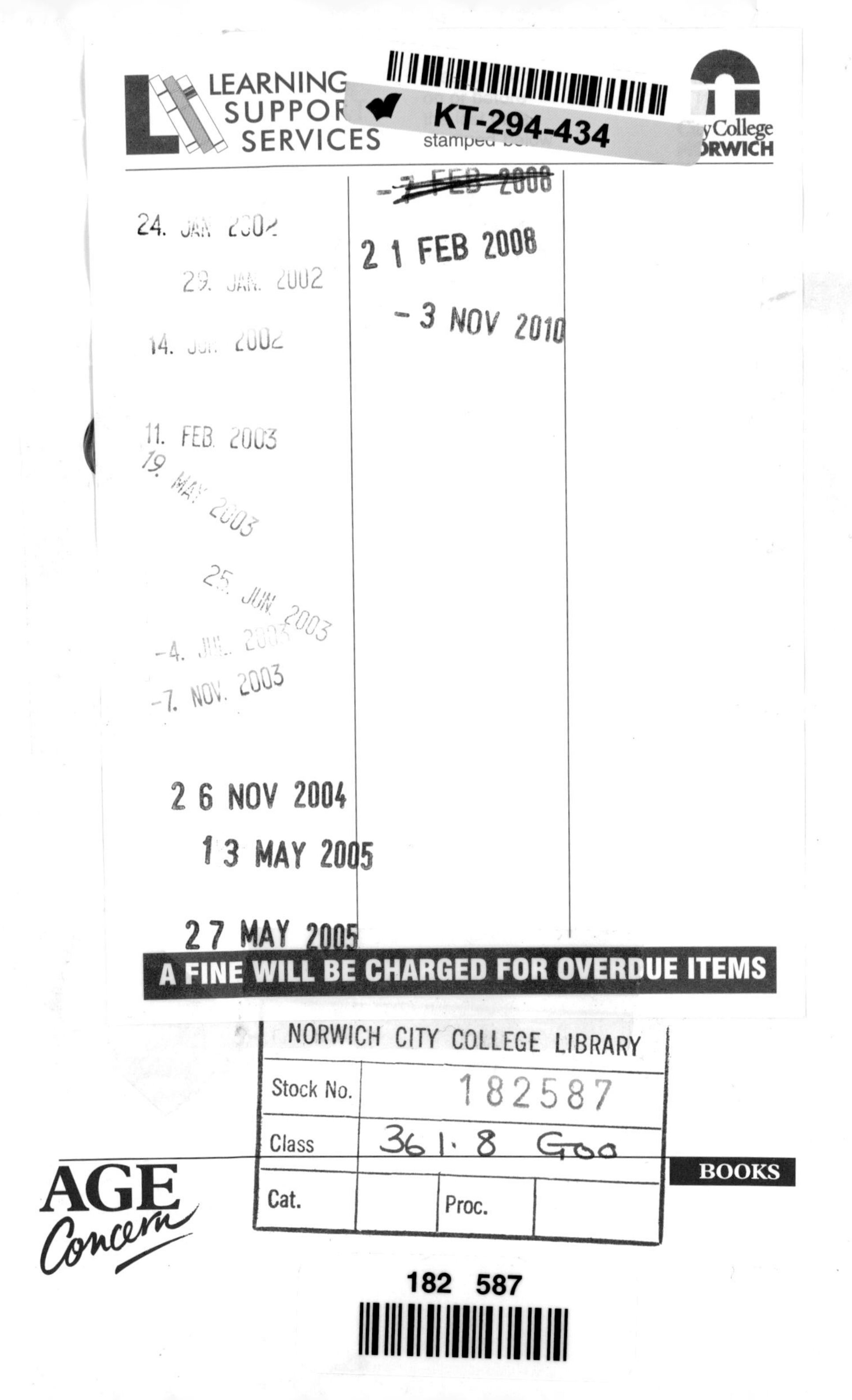
LEARNING SUPPORT SERVICES
KT-294-434
City College NORWICH
-7 FEB 2008
24. JAN 2002
21 FEB 2008
29. JAN. 2002
-3 NOV 2010
14. JUN. 2002
11. FEB. 2003
19. MAY 2003
25. JUN. 2003
-4. JUL. 2003
-7. NOV. 2003
26 NOV 2004
13 MAY 2005
27 MAY 2005
A FINE WILL BE CHARGED FOR OVERDUE ITEMS
NORWICH CITY COLLEGE LIBRARY
Stock No. 182587
Class 361.8 Goo
Cat.
Proc.
AGE Concern
BOOKS
182 587

Published by Age Concern England
1268 London Road
London SW16 4ER

First published 2001

Editor Judith Wardman
Production Vinnette Marshall
Design and typesetting GreenGate Publishing Services
Printed in Great Britain by Bell & Bain Ltd, Glasgow

A catalogue record for this book is available from the British Library.

ISBN 0-86242-340-6

Bulk orders

Age Concern England is pleased to offer customised editions of all its titles to UK companies, institutions or other organisations wishing to make a bulk purchase. For further information, please contact the Publishing Department at the address on this page. Tel: 020 8765 7200. Fax: 020 8765 7211. Email: books@ace.org.uk.

Contents

About the author

Alan Goodenough was the training manager of a large local authority social services department for 14 years. He is now a freelance writer and consultant, and tutors for the Open University. For the past six years, he has also been a voluntary carer.

Acknowledgements

My thanks are due to Sue Riches, from Suffolk Social Services, Clem le May and Jacqui Martin, from Suffolk Carers Ltd, and Pat Wilson, from the Suffolk NVQ Consortium, whose time, technical expertise and experience proved an invaluable aid in compiling this guide. My thanks also go to Lesley Bell, for wise advice and counsel, and to Teresa Goodenough, whose quiet support and encouragement, as always, proved invaluable.

Glossary

Care workers are paid to work in the caring services. They are sometimes called 'care assistants' or 'home carers'. **Voluntary carers** look after friends and relatives without pay.

The **Health Service** (or **NHS**) provides care and treatment in hospitals, and in the community (your GP's surgery, for instance, is a 'primary care' service within the NHS). The boundaries between health care provided by the NHS and social care provided by local authorities (see below) are sometimes rather blurred, so that older people and others may 'fall into the cracks' between each service (NHS Plan 2000). A number of recent initiatives (such as the care trusts mentioned below) plan to fill these gaps.

Local authorities All social services and social work departments (in Scotland) are part of a local authority. Most government documents refer to local authorities as 'councils', which is probably the way that you know them too. County Councils still provide social services in England, though there are also 'unitary' authorities in England, Wales and Scotland that provide both social services and housing services (amongst others). Social services in Northern Ireland are provided by combined health and social services trusts.

Health authorities probably fund most of the health services provided in your area. Increasingly, they fund the development of community services in conjunction with social services. Health authorities also 'plan, develop, and monitor' services provided by GPs, dentists, retail pharmacists, and opticians.

Primary care groups (or **PCGs**) plan and 'commission' health services for local areas in England. All GPs, social services and local 'lay' community interests are represented on the boards of primary care groups. By 2004, all primary care groups are expected to have become **primary care trusts** (or **PCTs**): ie, they will provide some of the community services they currently commission.

Care trusts will bring together the provision of health and social services into one organisation.

National Required Standards (or **NRSs**) are used to monitor and inspect the standards of care provided in residential care homes, and, very soon, in domiciliary care services as well. The advantage of having national standards, used extensively in the health service too, is that they set baselines for good care practice (so that no service should fall below that baseline), making it less likely that people living in one part of the country will not receive as good a service as people living somewhere else (what's often called the 'postcode lottery').

'For-profit' and **'not-for-profit' organisations** Most publicly funded services are provided by 'not-for-profit' organisations. These organisations cannot sell the services they offer, and any fees they charge go to offset their costs, or are passed on to other organisations (such as government departments). 'For-profit' organisations are just that: they can sell the services they offer at a profit. Their profits help create a 'return' on whatever capital they put up to start, maintain, or expand the business. For-profit organisations are generally in the 'private' sector, for example, private residential care homes.

Purchasing or **'commissioning'** a service (and 'commissioning' is probably the term you'll see most frequently used) means setting out the specification for that service, and, of course, setting out the price that the 'commissioner' is prepared to pay for it. Commissioners plan for the future as well as the present (what's called strategic planning). There are three steps involved in making any strategic plan: first, identify where you are now; second, decide where you want to be; and third, develop a plan which will move you from your current position to your future vision (RCN, 1998).

Providers are the organisations that deliver the service that commissioners have specified and paid for. Care workers are generally employed by provider services.

Introduction

This is a guide for those who care for older people. It's written for people who are care workers, but has much to say to people who care voluntarily. It's meant to help you find your way around health and welfare services for older people. It lets you know how those services work, and how to contact the right person when you need them. As many readers will know from their own experience, the services provided for older people come from a variety of different organisations, very few of which are found under the same roof. To make things harder still, many of these organisations have their own ways of deciding whom they can help, which means that older people often need someone who can open all these doors on their behalf.

There's a brief explanation of why services are broken up or 'fragmented' in this way in the section below headed 'The organisation of services'. Fortunately, there are developments designed to pull these services together, for example, the NHS and Community Care Act 1990, the Health Act 1999, the joint planning, purchase and inspection of health and social services, the NHS Plan 2000, and the Health and Social Care Bill 2001. You'll find these developments described in some detail later on. But this book is written now because:

- it's very important that care workers feel part of the caring 'team', whether or not they have 'professional' qualifications, and they can't do that without information – care workers can do a much better job of putting over the needs of the person they are caring for once they know whom to ask for the right kinds of help;
- it's just as important that older people don't 'fall through the net' because neither they nor their carers know where and how to get the right kinds of help. Though it's all too easy to 'take over' and make decisions older people should be making for themselves, there are still plenty of occasions when they need someone who can help to put their needs and views across. They are more likely to get the right kind of help when they need it if they or their care

workers know something about who does what, where to find them, and the sorts of help they should be asking for.

You might be wondering what we mean by 'older people'. Age alone is no guide to anyone's needs. We all know people who are old in years but still lead amazingly full and active lives. When Professor Laslett first used the phrase 'Third Age', he meant to get away from the notion that anyone over the age of 65 and retired was somehow frail and decrepit. The 'Third Agers' we have in mind may need a little help, but help of the sort that lets them lead full and independent lives, ideally in their own homes.

Some objectives

The book has three broad objectives:

1 To help identify all those people, 'professionals' and others, who can help you care for older people you work with.
2 To help you recognise the very important contribution you as a care worker make to the caring team.
3 To help you understand what services there are for older people, why they work in the way(s) they do, and what they can and cannot do.

You'll find 'Activities' in each chapter of this book. Most of them ask you to put something into your own words, or to think how what you've read might apply to people, or to write down ways of doing things in your own work setting. Activities are there to help you understand and remember what might at first sound like a complicated set of ideas. Putting something in your own words makes most things easier to understand. You'll have a much better chance of remembering what you've learned if you've thought through how those ideas affect the people you're working with. Usually there will be some clues or 'memory joggers' to help you think each Activity through.

ACTIVITY 1

Measuring our objectives

- Try to re-write the objectives above in your own words. You'll find some blank sheets bound into the back of this book in case that helps you to make notes, or you can use your own notebook. At the end of Chapter 3, we'll ask for your opinion on how well the book met its three objectives.

1

2

3

Who is this book for?

Because it describes 'community' services, this guide will help staff in services that are community-based, such as residential homes and nursing homes, and any form of home care or domiciliary services. There may be auxiliary nursing staff who find the guide of help. Staff in residential care homes will find it helps them understand how staff outside the homes can work alongside them in managing a resident's care plan. Staff in voluntary organisations may find it helps them to understand which of the 'statutory' services can best help someone in their care.

Many of those we want to read this guide will be relatively new in post, and it will also help those who are just at the start of a training course. More experienced care workers may find the book helps update or refresh their knowledge. If you're simply a little bewildered by some of the roles and responsibilities of staff who work in the health or welfare services, or if you're wondering how best to get help for an older person in your care, then whatever kind of care you provide, this guide should help you.

How can I use this book?

Unlike novels, you won't lose the plot by not reading this guide from cover to cover. If one section seems particularly relevant to something you need to know, then that may be the place you need to start. What we do want you to do is to read the book in full at some time (not necessarily all at once). The face of health and welfare services has changed so rapidly in recent years that you may get something wrong if you rely on single sections of the book, and not on the book as a whole.

Using the book as a basis for further study

Some of you may be thinking of going on to further study, such as Scottish or National Vocational Qualifications (S/NVQs) in Care at Levels 2 and 3. Parts of this guide may help you find the 'underpinning knowledge' you need for S/NVQs; it will be useful for other study programmes and courses too.

You'll find some references to individual S/NVQ units as you read through the guide; this should help you pick out any evidence you need (the references are in italic type). Even if you're not yet registered for S/NVQs, keep any notes you make (including the notes you make on the Activities), because these notes should help you to build up the 'portfolio' of evidence you'll need to complete any Scottish or National Vocational Qualification. *The whole guide is relevant to S/NVQ Care Level 2 Unit CL1, 'Promote effective communication and relationships'.* Please note that the Care Level Two Standards are currently being revised.

The organisation of services

You will have read that services for older people are provided by a number of different agencies ('agency' is one of those blanket words and stands for any organisation providing services). In other words, services for older people are relatively 'fragmented', that is, those services are provided by a variety of agencies with rather different ways of doing things and very different ways of raising funds.

This section will help you begin to understand why that fragmentation has come about. A good starting point is to divide the agencies providing services to older people into three broad categories, or sectors: the voluntary sector; the independent sector; and the public or statutory or state sector. If that sounds a little confusing, then think about a map you've seen that shows you several different countries. Each country has its own characteristics, but it probably has a lot in common with its neighbours, like the same kind of climate, or similar problems in feeding or educating its people. So it is with the three sectors. Each sector has much in common with the others (even if they don't always see eye to eye); the difference comes in the way each sector is managed and financed, and in the responsibilities each has towards the other. As you'll see later on, the way each sector finds and funds its work controls some very important decisions that staff in those sectors have to make, such as how much they charge for particular services. Let's look briefly at each of the three sectors.

The voluntary sector

Amongst the 'voluntaries' are large national organisations or networks like SCOPE, Age Concern, Crossroads and the Salvation Army (to name but a few). At the other end of the scale are relatively small organisations that might, for example, be responsible for just one residential home. Some voluntary organisations have been in existence for a very long time. Some are very large employers, but many depend as much or more on people who give their time voluntarily, like a committee of unpaid trustees. Many have charitable status, which means they aren't allowed to make a profit. The characteristic all 'voluntaries' share is that, to some extent, they have to make up their income by money raised directly from the public through, say, street collections or appeals in the press or on television. That means some services might be very difficult for a voluntary organisation to fund without outside help (since some 'causes' aren't very popular with the giving public). Nowadays, much of that outside help comes from providing services that other organisations are prepared to pay for, so that many voluntary organisations are very dependent on money from central government or local councils. For some voluntary organisations, this may limit the freedom they once had to create new services in response to new needs.

The private or independent sector

Many residential care homes, and an increasing number of domiciliary or home care agencies are owned by private-sector companies. The one characteristic all private-sector organisations share is that they must make a profit, or at the very least must sell enough of whatever services they provide to cover their costs. Some older people buy services like residential care, cleaning or shopping direct from private-sector organisations without the need to go through anyone else (ie, they've gone direct to the company concerned without asking someone like a social worker to help make arrangements for them). At least theoretically, these people are exercising their right as 'consumers' to buy the service they want, from a company of their choice, at whatever price they are prepared to pay for it (much in the same way that many of us make choices, say, about the kinds of clothes we buy, or the make of car we drive). They are, in effect, subsidising the cost of providing similar services for people who cannot afford to pay full cost for them. The difficulty many older people experience when care is compared to other products we use as consumers is that they can't exercise the same kind of choice when buying care as they might when buying, say, a pair of shoes. Either they can't afford to pay the full cost of any care they need, or they are not informed or supported enough to 'shop around' until they find the service they most wish to use (always assuming they live in an area where there are several similar services to choose from). Many private-sector organisations have to compete for the contracts that public-sector organisations give to reduce the cost of services for older people who cannot afford to pay 'full cost'. If contract prices are driven down (since purchasers will often look for the best quality at the best price they can get), then the risk is that some care-home beds will be lost at a time when demand for those beds continues to rise.

The public, state or 'statutory' sector

This divides into two main sections: health services provided the National Health Service (NHS) and social services provided by local authorities, that is, town, borough and county councils, and unitary authorities. Only in Northern Ireland have health and social services been combined into regional boards.

Both health and social services are part of what we now call the 'welfare state'. Often included in the welfare state are the various forms of welfare benefits (including the state retirement pension, Income Support, the Minimum Income Guarantee, Attendance Allowance etc), administered by the Benefits Agency (or the Social Security Agency in Northern Ireland). Much of the money public-sector organisations spend comes directly from the public purse (either from the money central government raises in taxation or, to a much lesser extent, for local authorities, from the Council Tax householders pay, or the property rates paid in Northern Ireland). Another feature of all public-sector agencies is that they must answer to, or consult, local people about the quality and content of services they provide.

Spending on all those services that make up the welfare state is now the largest single item of government expenditure. What has markedly changed in the last ten years or so are the numbers of services that social services/social work departments provide themselves, such as residential care homes or home care services. For example, whilst around half of all residential care homes for older people in England and Wales were staffed and managed by local authorities in the late 1980s, not much more than 20 per cent are still in local authority control (though the change has not been quite so drastic in Scotland and Northern Ireland). From being 'providers' of services themselves, social services departments have moved to being 'purchasers' and inspectors of services other agencies provide. There have also been some very significant changes in the way that health services are organised; you'll find these described in Chapter 2.

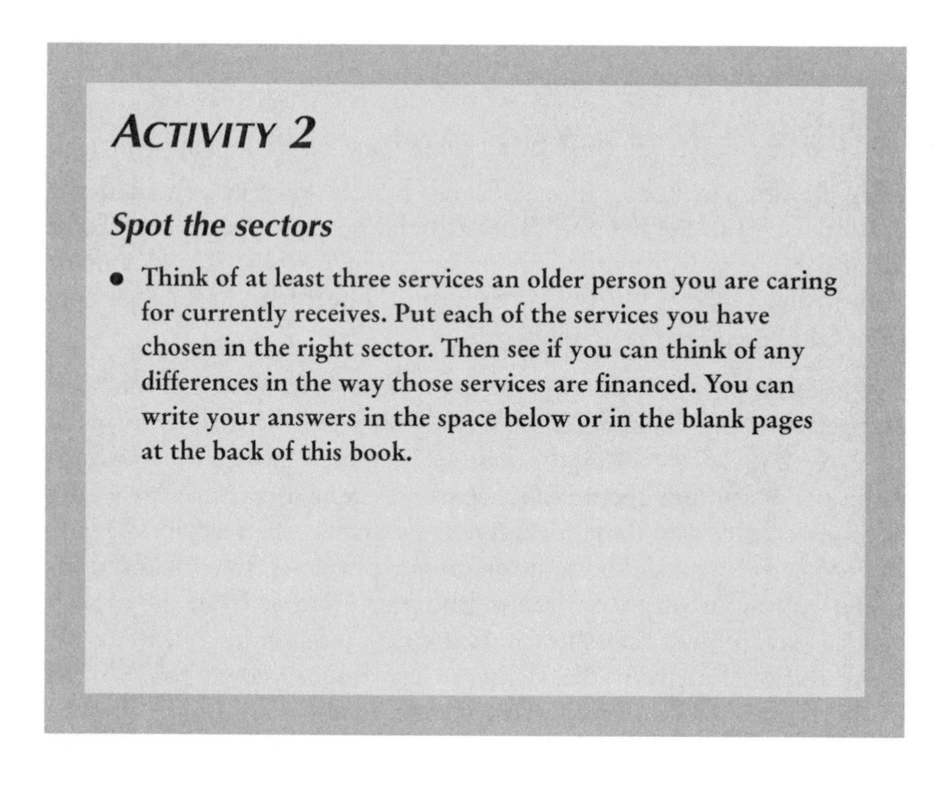

Activity 2

Spot the sectors

- Think of at least three services an older person you are caring for currently receives. Put each of the services you have chosen in the right sector. Then see if you can think of any differences in the way those services are financed. You can write your answers in the space below or in the blank pages at the back of this book.

The legal background

The following paragraphs will help S/NVQ candidates find the underpinning knowledge they need to 'evidence' Care Level 2 Unit Z1, 'Contribute to the protection of individuals from abuse'.

In very general terms, all the community care services available to older people are subject to the law, and many are governed by Acts of Parliament that set out the powers that service has, or in some way set out what staff providing those services can do 'within the law.' Some public-sector services are called 'statutory' services because they are governed by parliamentary statute (usually an Act of Parliament). There isn't space in this guide to describe all the legislation that applies to older people's services (not forgetting that Scotland and Northern Ireland have their own legal systems, and there are laws that only apply to those countries, and occasionally, laws that only apply to England or to Wales). But, like every other citizen, you must obey and uphold the law that applies in whatever part of the country you work in. That doesn't mean you have to memorise a lot of complicated legal language (that, after all, is what managers and solicitors are paid to do); it does mean you should have in the back of your mind that the law – whatever its imperfections – is there to protect the people you care for. S/NVQ candidates working on Unit Z1 must show they 'know and understand' the legislation affecting whatever group of service users they are working with.

What you may be surprised to discover is that there is no single Act of Parliament that protects vulnerable old people; different Acts apply to different offences. All the laws relating to criminal behaviour in general apply equally to older people. For example, it could be illegal – or abusive – to limit someone's freedom to make their own choices, for instance by cutting back the amount of money a person is entitled to have each week without their genuine consent. The law quite specifically protects people with mental health problems or learning disabilities from sexual exploitation, ill treatment and neglect. There are also legal protections for people who cannot look after their own financial affairs (which may involve their giving someone else an 'Enduring Power of Attorney').

As those of you working in residential homes will probably know, there are very specific powers to regulate and inspect care homes and nursing homes throughout the United Kingdom (see the next section). The Department of Health has produced National Required Standards (NRSs) which all residential and nursing homes are required to meet (The National Required Standards for Residential and Nursing Homes). There is also health and safety legislation, the regulation of employment agencies, and employment laws (such as the Working Time Directive) that protect you as an employee.

What you should always remember is that when older people are at risk of being hurt in any way, there is never an excuse for keep-

ing quiet. If you have any suspicion that an older person is being abused, you should always report it to someone who can do something about it. Most local authorities have procedures for protecting older people thought to have been abused. Many of the organisations you work for will have procedures for dealing with 'elder abuse' (especially if their services are contracted to a local authority or NHS trust). Don't delay if the situation is complicated, or if you can't quite 'firm up' what you suspect may be happening. Any manager in the caring services should know where they can go for further advice.

ACTIVITY 3

The legal framework

- **Why do you think carers should have some knowledge of the law? Use the space below to write down your answers.**

Registration and inspection

All residential homes for older people in the private and voluntary sectors, whatever their size, must register with their local authority (ie, social services departments in England and Wales, social work departments in Scotland, and the health and social service boards in Northern Ireland). 'Dual registered' homes, where some residents need care from appropriately qualified nursing staff, and nursing homes must also register with their local health authority. A registered home must meet certain minimum standards. Local authority inspectors (sometimes called 'standards' or 'registration' officers) visit every registered home in their area, and homes that fail to meet 'registration standards' could be forced to close. Health authorities have similar powers to inspect and, if necessary, to close nursing homes.

Regulation and inspection responsibilities are set to change between 2001 and 2002. All homes, including local authority homes, or the 'statutory' homes in Northern Ireland, are to be regularly inspected by staff from the National Commission for Care Standards (in England). Different arrangements apply in other parts of the United Kingdom. Homes with fewer than four residents might not be inspected, but they are required to register with their local authority. The National Commission, which is part of the Department of Health, takes on what have been local authority and health authority responsibilities for registration and inspection in April 2002. For the first time, many domiciliary services will be inspected too, including any service that 'contracts' with a local authority, or a care trust. These new arrangements should even out some of the variations in inspection practice from one authority to another. The National Commission will apply the same standards to every part of England.

Anyone, including residents and their families, who is worried about something they think is going wrong in any residential home can complain to the registration and inspections unit of their local authority – the number is usually in the phone book. Though it's never easy to 'blow the whistle' on your colleagues, staff working in any service to older people are also entitled to raise their concerns about poor practice, especially if there is the slightest hint that a resident or other service user is being abused. If you ever find yourself in this position, and cannot share your worries with your own line manager (for whatever reason), then speak to the person who is next senior to your manager. Many organisations have worked out special sets of procedures to protect staff who 'whistle blow' in this way (see page 78). If local authority inspectors, or care standards 'commissioners', visit a home, or anywhere else where you work, then you're also entitled to speak to them in private. Residents and other service users have the same rights to privacy (Section **48** [4] of the NHS and Community Care Act; see below).

The National Health Service and Community Care Act 1990

To understand this Act, you also need to understand some of the thinking behind it. Much of what is now the 'NHS and Community Care Act' was based on a report by Sir Roy Griffiths. The background to his work was a very critical report from the Audit Commission on the rapidly rising costs of making (the pre-1993) social security payments to older people living in residential homes; many of them, the Commission argued, could have stayed in their own homes with appropriate support. The Commission was equally concerned about people who remained in psychiatric hospitals and hospitals for people with learning disabilities but who could, again with support, be living 'in the community'.

Some of Sir Roy's recommendations were that:

- Money spent on helping people pay for residential care should be diverted into services that would help them stay in their own homes – there had to be a test of whether people wanting help to pay their fees really needed residential care (ie, they would have to have an assessment of their care needs, usually made by a social worker).
- There should be a separation between the 'purchasing' and 'provision' of care which would lead to services being 'needs-led', not 'service-driven'. If that sounds a little complicated, then think of the conflicts of interest that might arise if someone making assessments (ie, the 'purchaser') also works for an agency 'providing' services to older people – service users might not be getting the best available service *for them* if assessments were 'driven' by the need to keep existing services stocked with customers.
- Assessment responsibilities should be brought together in one post, rather than different people in different places making individual assessments of the same service users' needs. A 'care manager', who would usually be employed by a social services/social work department, would make an initial assessment, and contact other services as appropriate. The care manager would be expected to recommend, and possibly to purchase, the best available service for the person in need.

- There should be a better co-ordinated, or 'seamless', service, with a strong emphasis on health and social services/social work departments working more closely together, making it easier for older and disabled people to get the right services to support them at home.

What relevant parts of the NHS and Community Care Act say (put very briefly) is that:

- If anyone appeared to be in need of community care (which had, of course, to include residential care – see Sir Roy's first recommendation above – but generally meant services provided in the person's own home), then the local authority had to assess their needs, and on the basis of that assessment, 'decide whether [those] needs call for the provision by them of any ... services' (Section **47** [1]).
- Local authorities had to set up complaints procedures for anyone who felt that their needs had not been properly assessed, and/or that a service they needed had not been provided for them (Sections **50** [7b] and **52** [5b]).
- Every local authority had to prepare a plan for community care services that were going to be provided in their area, and they had to consult health authorities, housing authorities, and voluntary organisations when they came to prepare that plan (Sections **46** and **52** [5a]). *In practice, these are known as 'community care plans', and are published once a year.*

One of the most important things for you to remember about the NHS and Community Care Act is that it gives any older or disabled person the right to ask for an assessment of whatever help they think they need. (This is usually known as a 'community care assessment'.) Local authorities can set what are called 'eligibility criteria' to restrict the way they define someone's need for services, but no one can be denied that service if they meet those criteria. But a tragedy of our age is that so many people go without because they haven't asked for help; please encourage any older or disabled person to use the legal right this Act gives them to ask for an assessment (and to complain if they think they've been treated unfairly).

The Act also said a great deal about the creation of NHS 'trusts', and you'll find these referred to on page 51. Care management (along with 'purchasing and provision') is something described at much greater length on page 4 onwards.

Voluntary carers – as distinct from the people they care for – also have a right to ask for their needs to be assessed (under the Carers [Recognition and Services] Act 1995, and, since April 2001, under the Carers and Disabled Children Act 2000). You'll find this right referred to again on page 36.

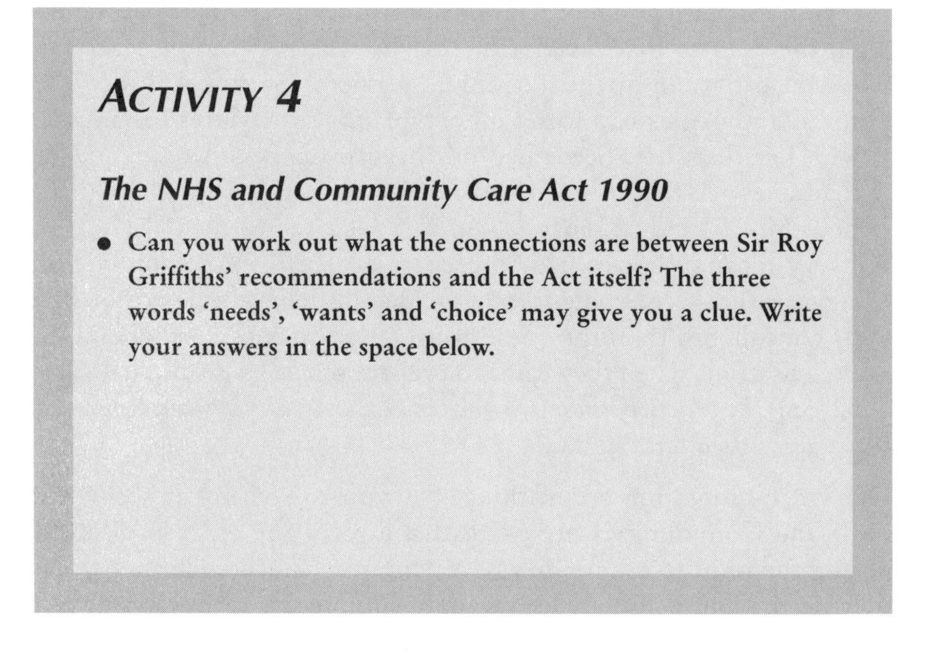

Activity 4

The NHS and Community Care Act 1990

- **Can you work out what the connections are between Sir Roy Griffiths' recommendations and the Act itself? The three words 'needs', 'wants' and 'choice' may give you a clue. Write your answers in the space below.**

Which leads you into the first chapter of this guide, where we look at care management, care planning and review.

1 Care management, care planning and review

Asking for help

You will have seen from the Introduction that getting help to an older person in need usually means that person has to 'go through' someone else: they must either know the right door to knock on, or someone has to help them find that door. We know from research (for example, Barner et al, 1982) that older people are more likely than many other groups to need help in 'referring' themselves to any of the welfare services.

ACTIVITY 5

Asking for help

- **See if you can complete the following sentence for yourself. Older people might have difficulty asking for help because they don't know what to ask for; they don't speak English as a first language; they are frightened of ...**

This chapter as a whole will help S/NVQ candidates find the underpinning knowledge they need to evidence Care Level 2 Units CL1, 'Promote effective communication and relationships', and Y1, 'Enable individuals to manage their domestic and personal resources'.

Working with people who pay for their own care

When you read through the Griffiths recommendations on pages xix–xx, you may have spotted one group of people who can refer themselves for help without having anyone make an independent assessment of their needs. These are people who choose to pay for their own residential care or for their own home care. In other words, they are exercising their right as consumers to purchase something they want to buy. Local authorities are under no obligation to arrange residential care for people who have more than £18,500 in capital, provided they are capable of making those arrangements for themselves. It's still possible, for example, to enter a private residential home by making your own arrangements direct with the home's proprietor, providing that you have sufficient capital to see you through at least the first part of your stay there. Charging policies for different services are described at the end of this chapter; something important for you to note at this stage is that people who pay the full charge for their own services are not necessarily immensely wealthy. Many care home residents have been obliged to sell quite modest properties to pay for their care. You might also be working with people who are using an Attendance Allowance to buy in some form of personal care, or people who are considered to need help only with shopping and cleaning (something most local authority home care services no longer provide) and buy these services direct from an independent home care agency, or a 'not-for-profit' organisation in the voluntary sector.

Some of the people who purchase care in this way will be relatively isolated (which is partly why your attention is being drawn to their needs). They may not see their doctor (GP) very often, and their 'case' may have been closed by social services because their care needs are less 'intensive' than those of other service users. As you'll see later on, one of the difficulties facing social services/social work departments anywhere in the country is that they find it harder to provide the sorts of 'preventive' services that keep in touch with older people whose health or personal circumstances are likely to deteriorate. Carers (paid or voluntary) often find themselves being the most important link between the person they care for and the outside world of caring services. It's very important that you use that link to alert, say, your manager or the person's GP to any change in a service user's condition that might suggest they need some additional help (though please take care to put your referral in a way the person concerned would respect, and remember any special needs, such as the religious or dietary preferences of people from minority groups).

Making choices and direct payments

Of course, we shouldn't assume that older people are somehow incapable of choosing the kind of care that suits them best. The best way to help someone make a decision for themselves is to set out what their options are, being as fair and balanced as possible in the way you do that, and then to wait as long as it takes for the person concerned to make their decision. That may be easier said than done, especially if you're very close to the person, but there's often a fine dividing line between protecting someone from harm, and undermining their independence.

The well-intentioned ease with which an older person's life can be taken over is recognised in one sense by a government initiative, ie, 'direct payments'. The first direct payments were made to disabled people under the age of 65, using the Community Care (Direct Payments) Act of 1996. From February 2000, direct payments have been available to older people, and from April 2001 to voluntary carers (under the Carers and Disabled Children Act 2000). With direct payments, older people, for instance, can be given a cash sum equivalent to the cost of providing services they need, on the understanding that they make their own arrangements to buy in those services; buy them from independent and voluntary organisations (not from local authorities or, in time, from care trusts); employ their own carers; and spend the money given them 'appropriately and cost-effectively'. Disabled people using the direct payments scheme may have already employed some of you (though the implementation of direct payments nationally has been patchy). Friends and family can be 'employed' by someone using direct payments, providing they do not live in the same household as the person they are caring for, and there are no other means of care available. Someone using direct payments can also have a mix of services, some of which they buy themselves, whilst at the same time other services continue to be provided by the local authority or a care trust. 'Direct payments promote independence ... by offering opportunities for rehabilitation, for education, leisure and employment for people in need of community care' (Department of Health, 1999). Direct payments cannot be used to buy in services from the National Health Service. If a local authority normally charges for its services, such as the charges made for home care, for instance, those charges will be deducted from the direct payments.

Care management

'Care management' is largely the responsibility of social services departments (or their equivalents in Scotland and Northern Ireland). You'll remember that Sir Roy Griffiths suggested that anyone in need of community care was more likely to get a full and balanced assessment of their needs if their initial assessment was made by a single worker who could assess for several needs at the same time (rather than several different workers, sometimes from different sections of the same department, each acting on their own independent assessment of what that person required). Service users, it was argued, shouldn't be left with unmet needs because no one sees them as 'whole people'; if one worker assesses them only for one set of needs, such as home care, that worker could overlook another equally important set of needs, such as mobility aids.

Care managers were meant to look at someone's 'wants and needs' without being 'driven' by the need to supply services provided by their own agency. They were also encouraged to use resources in the local community, especially if that helped someone to keep in touch with people they knew (though the enthusiasm local people sometimes have for helping their older neighbours is something few care managers have really built on).

However, you need to note that guidance from the Department of Health (1998) suggests that it can be helpful if an older person with very complex needs is assessed by different workers with different kinds of specialist skills (though someone still needs to act as lead, or 'trusted', assessor in order to keep the assessment process properly co-ordinated).

Where do I find a care manager?

In social services and social work departments, and in health and social services boards (or the NHS trusts that are replacing the boards in Northern Ireland). Care management is one of those terms that often stands for a way of working rather than an actual job title. Some social services have staff they call care managers; others have staff doing a similar job but with a different job title (though the likelihood is that those care managers who hold a professional qualification will have trained as social workers). You may find care managers, for example, called Care Co-ordinators, Community Care Managers, Community Care Practitioners, Support Service Workers or Support Service Managers. Many work in something called an 'adult' service, or adult team. Not all are found in borough/county council offices; some are based in hospitals, or even in GP surgeries. A few will work from home, using 'caller points' (often in council buildings) for anyone wishing to contact them.

Anyone wanting a community care assessment should start by contacting their local social services/social work department. If you can't find their number in the phone book, then the Citizens Advice Bureau, the local library and many voluntary organisations such as Age Concern will always help. Alternatively, a GP, practice nurse, district nurse, Macmillan nurse or hospital or hospice staff can 'refer' someone for assessment (providing they have that person's permission to do so).

ACTIVITY 6

Knocking on the care manager's door

- **Very few older people refer themselves to social services departments. They are referred by their GP, by other agencies or by their family or friends. Do carers have a role in helping**

people overcome their fear of 'officialdom'? Jot down your answer below.

How are community care assessments carried out?

This section and the section on 'How can I tell whether an assessment has been done properly?' (pages 10–11) will help provide the underpinning knowledge required for S/NVQ Care Level 2 Units W2, 'Contribute to the ongoing support of clients and others significant to them', W3, 'Support individuals experiencing a change in their care requirements and provision', and Z8, 'Support individuals when they are distressed'.

Community care assessments are often carried out in the service user's own home, especially if one of the points at issue is how well they can look after themselves, though many assessments are made in hospitals, as part of the arrangements needed to discharge someone home with adequate supports. Some departments use a list of questions, many of which are designed to help the assessor discover what the service user can do for themselves; what kinds of help they already receive; and who provides that help. The importance of checklists, though they look daunting, is that every care manager using them asks the same set of questions. Like every other 'public servant', care managers must be seen to be acting fairly in the way they allocate resources; asking everyone they assess the same questions means that all prospective service users start from a roughly level playing field. You'll probably find that assessment forms have been replaced by some form of computerised recording system now, since this makes it far easier for most departments to manage, and keep track of the demand for their services.

There's also a very important provision in the National Service Framework for Older People (2001). By April 2002 a 'single assessment process' must be used for any health or social care an older person receives (National Service Framework, 2001), ie, a single 'trusted assessor' makes that assessment, using an agreed process and format, on behalf of both health and social care services involved in that person's care. Now why is this so important? If you think back to the very beginning of this book, you'll have learned that the services many older people need come not just from one, but from a variety of 'agencies' (from the NHS, from social service and social work departments, and from the independent sector). No one starts down any of these 'complex care pathways' (National Service Framework) without assessment(s). Duplicating these assessments (and sadly, that still happens) is a waste of everybody's time. Worse still, once information gets scattered over several storage systems, or once we allow assessment to focus on one set of needs at the expense of others (which assessments confined to the needs of just one agency invariably do), the harder it becomes to see the 'whole person'. Lose sight of someone's individuality (of particular importance for people from diverse cultural backgrounds), and we may lose sight of what it is they want and need. Lose that, and we make it harder for older people to live independently, with dignity, in their own homes, putting them at risk of inappropriate admissions to hospital, or to a residential care home. 'Service provision [should be] person centred, regardless of professional and organisational boundaries' (National Service Framework, 2001).

If you're helping an older person prepare for their community care assessment (or any other form of assessment), then here are some issues that person might like to be thinking about before they meet the assessor; but please read through the whole of the next section and Activity 7 before you put any of these suggestions to them.

The person concerned might think of asking for:

- changes to the home and/or equipment to help them manage in their home;
- someone to help with personal care (eg, bathing);
- a meal (or meals) delivered;

- a regular (or occasional) break for someone who cares for them voluntarily;
- a discussion about temporary or permanent residential care;
- the chance to talk to someone about a problem they have;
- information about what is available and its costs.

If you know of anything else that's important to the person concerned, then add that to the list. Encourage the person being assessed to think of anything that would make their lives a little easier. Help them to say what it is they really want, as distinct from what they think the assessor wants to hear from them. The easiest thing in the world is to 'slot someone in' to a service that already exists. A distinguishing mark of age-related discrimination is the assumption that older people must 'make do' with existing services, whether or not that service fully meets their needs. Don't forget that health and social care planning systems have been localised (as you'll see when you come to read about primary care groups, for instance) precisely because it's easier to create a service that responds to individual need when services are planned at local level. 'Too frequently people are fitted to services rather than services fitted to people's needs' (A Quality Strategy for Social Care, 2000).

By and large, you'll find assessors very reluctant to do anything that might make an older person more dependent on services than they already are. If someone can still do something for themselves, however slowly or awkwardly, then many assessors would prefer to let them retain that degree of independence (with the assistance, perhaps, of a suitable aid, such as grab handles or a raised toilet seat).

Many assessors will want to speak to an older person alone. If this makes you feel at all uneasy, then think of things this way. An assessor's first responsibility is to the older person being assessed. They have to get a view of the world as that person sees it. The likelihood is that most assessors would be very pleased if you offered to leave them alone for a while with the older person (this might be the time to make a cup of tea or coffee, for example).

Don't forget that voluntary carers now have a right to have their needs assessed too, and assessors must always take note of this. There will be times when an older person needs your help in putting something across, though it's a wise idea to have agreed and rehearsed what you're going to say for that person before the assessment begins (it saves any distress afterwards, as well as being far more respectful to the person concerned). Remember that your role is to help the older person speak for themselves, so that what you say, for the most part, is what you agreed you would say before the assessment began. Remember too that experienced assessors always know when someone is being a little 'economical with the truth'.

ACTIVITY 7

When to speak out, and when to keep quiet

- **Try to imagine yourself being present during an older person's community care assessment. Write a few lines in your own words about what you might want to say, and when you would say it. Use the blank pages at the back of this book if that's easier for you.**

Are some assessments triggered automatically?

If an older person is waiting on discharge from hospital, then the probability is that they'll be offered a community care assessment or re-assessment (to help decide, and put in place, the help they'll need once home, or to help them look at options and alternatives if they need care away from home). Hospital-based assessments are likely to be made by a member of the hospital-based social work team, though they'll probably hand over whatever responsibilities they had for making sure the care package is working properly within a short time of the service user leaving hospital (like many hospital staff, they find it difficult not to make the next patient due for discharge the focus of their attention). Don't forget that if someone needs help to pay for particular services (such as home care, or care home places), they'll have to declare what money they have coming in each week/month, and what assets they own. Local authorities always hold such information in confidence, though no one should be pressured into revealing anything about their financial circumstances if they would rather pay the full cost of any service they receive.

How can I tell whether an assessment has been done properly?

Here are some 'pointers' that should help you. A good assessor will:

- 'empower' both the user and their carer(s): inform fully, clarify their understanding of the situation and of the role of the assessor before going ahead;
- involve, rather than just inform, the user and their carer(s), making them feel they are full partners in the assessment;
- shed their 'professional' perspective: have an open mind and be prepared to learn;
- start from where the user and carers are, establish their existing level of knowledge and what hopes and expectations they have;
- be interested in the user and their carers as people;
- establish a suitable environment for the assessment, which ensures privacy, quiet and sufficient time;
- take time – build trust and understanding, and overcome the 'brief visitor' effect (which will usually take more than one visit);
- be sensitive, creative and imaginative in responding – users and carers may not know what is possible or available, and, for carers in particular, guilt and reticence may have to be overcome;
- consider social, emotional and relationship needs, as well as just practical needs and difficulties; pay particular attention to the quality of the relationship between the user and their carers;
- listen to and value the user's and carers' expertise or opinions, even if these run counter to the assessor's own values;

- present honest, realistic service options, identifying advantages and disadvantages and providing an indication of any delay or limitations in service delivery;
- not make assessment a 'battle' in which users and their carers feel they have to fight for services;
- balance all viewpoints;
- make certain everyone knows what has been agreed by the end of the review process, and are clear about review dates etc.

(Nolan and Caldock, 1996)

Do care managers always work for social services?

Mostly, but not always, since social services have the 'lead' responsibility for making community care assessments. 'Named' assessors can be appointed from other disciplines (eg, an experienced nurse, a community psychiatric nurse, or an occupational therapist). Social services departments cannot delegate their lead assessment responsibilities at present, though the Health and Social Care Bill 2001 may change this.

Is there a financial element in every community care assessment?

No, some people opt to pay in full for their own 'care package', though many local authorities make it a matter of policy to check on someone's entitlement to welfare benefits (eg, Attendance Allowance or Income Support) as part of every community care assessment. Far too many welfare benefits go unclaimed because older people are not aware they might be entitled to claim them. But no one has to pay anything for a community care assessment carried out by social services, or, in future, by a care trust.

Don't forget there are special financial provisions for people who are terminally ill. These are known as 'Special Rules'. They mean that someone who is terminally ill can receive benefits like the Disability Living Allowance, or Attendance Allowance, without having to wait through the usual 'qualifying' period (three months for DLA and six months for Attendance Allowance).

Can everyone ask for a copy of their community care assessment?

They may be given one automatically. If not, they have a right to see most of the information kept on file about them. The complication is (and this is more an explanation than an excuse) that some computer records may be difficult to interpret – they're meant to store statistics rather than information – and some people's circumstances change so rapidly that their care package needs constantly updating. However, users and their carer(s) can find it very helpful – and empowering – to have a written record of how their needs have been assessed.

What is a 'care package'?

Whatever arrangements for help and support are put in place after the community care assessment.

Can care managers arrange for the provision of health and housing services?

Social workers are not qualified medical practitioners and cannot exercise what's called a clinical judgement on the allocation of health service resources. Nor should they offer a medical opinion on the user's health. There are many examples of health and social services staff working together in the interests of older people (what the government calls a 'joined up' service); sadly, there are just as many occasions when co-operation goes badly wrong (which is why there are already successful 'partnerships' of health and social service staff working from the 'primary care team', or doctor's surgery; which is why health and social services have jointly invested in the planning and provision of services; and which is why the NHS Plan 2000 looks ahead to the joint provision of services through care trusts). Care managers should always involve health staff in the person's assessment, and will clearly need to do so once the single assessment process starts to work (National Service Framework for Older People, 2001). This is especially important if the person being assessed needs some form of nursing care.

Housing is also a service that English county councils, and Northern Irish health and social service boards do not provide (though most other local authorities do, and many are experimenting with 'one-stop shops' where housing, social services departments, and other services may share the same office buildings, and/or one receptionist can handle any enquiries). Unsafe housing (whoever owns the property) may also put an older person into high risk categories (see below) for the allocation of welfare services. Many local authorities are developing very sheltered housing schemes as an alternative to more traditional forms of residential care.

Eligibility criteria

As you saw on page xx, under the NHS and Community Care Act 1990, local authorities must assess everyone in need of community care, even if in some circumstances they choose not to provide some of the services the person needs. The problem is that many local authorities can afford to pay for less and less, and demand continues to grow. Some authorities have seen the demand for their services rise by seven or eight times the level it was in 1993, when the NHS and Community Care Act came fully into force. Over the ten years 1990–2000, there has also been an increase of something like a third in the numbers of people aged 85 and over (and whilst there are many fit and healthy people living well into their 80s, the over-85s do tend to need more help from community care services than younger people).

What are eligibility criteria?

Basically a way of restricting services to those 'whose need for them is greatest' (*Caring for People*, 1989), though many authorities also try to make sure their services go to older people at greatest risk, and those who are most dependent on outside help. The NHS also uses a form of eligibility criteria (known as continuing care criteria) when health authorities come to decide on the sorts of individual health care needs that qualify someone for such continuing health care services as care in an NHS contracted bed in a private nursing home, rehabilitation and recovery, or palliative care to the terminally ill (Age Concern Factsheet 37 *Hospital discharge arrangements and NHS continuing healthcare services*). Unfortunately, whilst there are encouraging signs that health authorities and social services departments are standardising criteria locally, across the country as a whole there are still considerable variations in the criteria that decide someone's eligibility for continuing health care, or local authority community care services. This leads to criticism, in the 'fair access to care service' proposals, for instance (*Modernising Social Services*, 1998), that the level of service older people receive differs widely in different parts of the country. The government is currently consulting on proposals that would standardise eligibility criteria and even out these variations in service levels. As Age Concern suggest, 'there is a clear need for national standards, so that older people have equal access to care, no matter where they live, and social services criteria for agreeing it are clear and reliable' (Kendra, 1997).

There's another equally serious downside to the way eligibility criteria are currently applied. Once a service is restricted to those in greatest need (remember the very beginning of this section), then people whose needs are not seen to be quite as urgent may not get any or all of the help they need, even if providing some form of service would prevent their condition from getting worse. Fortunately, there is (some) reason to hope that the importance of 'preventive' services will be given greater emphasis. Both 'intermediate care' and 'rehabilitation' (see pages 53–55) are important preventive services, since they help to break what the Audit Commission (*The Way to go Home: Rehabilitation and Remedial Services for Older People*, 2000) calls the 'vicious circle' of unnecessary admissions to residential homes, or unnecessary re-admissions of older people to hospital. The National Service Framework for Older People sets important targets for the development of intermediate care. (Some) funding for preventive services has also been provided as 'prevention grants', part of which has funded the 'short break' or 'respite' services for carers you could have experienced (though the Promoting Independence Grant that funded prevention grants was ended in April 2001). The new care trusts will also be expected to 'adopt one unified set of criteria that will cover all the user needs for which help will be provided' (*Guidance on the Health Act Section 31*, 2000).

How do eligibility criteria work?

Broadly speaking, in one of three ways:

1 By limiting the numbers of people getting particular services. Assessors using this system will be asked to rank the people they assess according to the severity or urgency of their needs. They might, for example, decide that someone has 'high needs', 'moderate needs' or 'low needs'. The likelihood is that people in the low-needs category will not get local authority help in organising, providing, or paying for any services that could be of benefit to them.
2 By limiting the cost of any services given. This system works by giving each older person *x* amount of any service they need, but spending more on those at greatest risk (up to whatever 'ceiling' the authority agrees). In other words, everyone gets something of what they may have asked for, but very few people get all of what they asked for (and sadly, some people will be denied domiciliary services if the cost of providing those services is more than their local authority would pay for residential care home places).
3 By limiting the types of service offered. This is where departments set a 'level' of service (eg, *x* hours of home care per week for people needing a certain level of help with daily living skills), but vary the level or type of care each person receives according, say, to how much care and support they receive from family and friends, and the willingness of family and friends to continue giving that care. With this system, a very isolated old person might continue to get help with shopping and cleaning, for example, if that need was important to them, whilst someone with help available from friends and family, though they might be in frailer health, could be refused a similar service; but, of course, the contribution that carers make to meeting someone's needs should always be recorded on their care plan.

You'll probably find that some authorities use a combination of these systems (it really is hard to set eligibility criteria); all this section does is to give you a very brief overview of how those criteria work in practice.

How do eligibility criteria affect my work with service users?

You may have found that the number of hours you are allocated to work with particular service users has changed in some way. Of course, people's dependency needs do change, but it is possible the hours were changed because your authority tightened its eligibility criteria (in which a new assessment is legally required).

Why do I need to know about them?

- As you probably thought when you read through 'How do eligibility criteria work?', eligibility criteria can be difficult to understand in practice. If someone you know has recently had a community care assessment and is still feeling puzzled by the outcome, knowing something about how eligibility criteria are applied in your area might help you give them a fuller explanation of what's happened.
- No one's needs stand still, or at least not for very long. If someone's condition deteriorates, they may become eligible for services they had previously been refused. Many people will be reluctant to ask again if they've already had help refused or have not been given all they might have hoped for. You'll be of greater help to such a person if you know something about the eligibility criteria used in your area (and you could be better prepared to 'advocate' on their behalf as well).
- Every older person has a right to complain if they think they've not been fairly treated by any public authority (see pages 77–78). It could be your responsibility to remind them of that right (especially if they think that eligibility criteria have not been correctly applied in their case).

Activity 8

Finding out about eligibility criteria

- **Where would you go to find out about eligibility criteria or the continuing care criteria used in the National Health Service? Jot down some good starting points below. Here are some clues to get you going: your line manager should know where the criteria for your area can be found, but if you are working on your own, try your authority's Community Care Plan, or the annual reports published each year by the NHS Trusts in your area – there should be copies in your public library.**

The individual care plan

Once an assessment has been done, using whatever criteria apply locally, the results of that assessment must be written into an individual care plan. Don't forget that a care plan is not quite the same as a community care assessment; the plan is the outcome of that assessment, since it puts in place the service someone requires. You'll already be familiar with some, at least, of the elements in a good care plan:

- **partnership** – between 'professionals', service users, and their carers (ie, everyone, especially professionals from different agencies, needs to be pulling in the same direction);
- clear lines of '**accountability**' – one named person should be responsible to the service user for putting their care plan into action;

- **responsiveness** – to what the service user wants and needs, without 'tramlining' them into services that happen to be there (when another service might be better for them), or involving them in conflicts between professional workers or their agencies;
- **access** – to a range of services (including the housing needs of service users and their relatives).
- **person-centred planning** – which makes the person being assessed more important than any of the problems with organisational 'boundaries' you read about earlier on. It also means that all health and social staff will have to make a very deliberate effort to find out just what older people think about the quality and value of any services they receive (National Service Framework for Older People, 2001).

More specifically, the care plan also needs to:

- be factually correct (it's disrespectful to misspell someone's name, for example);
- make clear statements about someone's wants, needs and preferences, without using 'jargon' words that service users or their carers may not understand;
- be very clear about who is going to do what, and when they are going to do it (especially if the older person concerned is waiting to leave hospital);
- name someone who is responsible for making sure that anything agreed in the plan is actually carried out;
- set an agreed time and date for the plan to be reviewed.

Service users should always have a written copy of their care plan. They should also be told, in writing, of any charges they may have to pay, and how they should pay those charges (where to buy their home care 'stamp', for example, or how to use any payment cards involved). Don't forget that no one can be said to have agreed their care plan if they're not absolutely clear how much they have to pay for the services involved.

The *NHS Continuing Care Notification Form* serves a similar function to social services care plans (generally for patients whose ongoing care needs will be met within the NHS).

ACTIVITY 9

Using the care plan

- Many of you will be working to at least one care plan, and probably to several (one for each of the people you work with). What is the importance of the care plan for you as a care worker? Look back to 'Why do I need to know about them?' for some extra clues. Try to write two or three sentences on the importance of care plans below, including a line or two on the importance of person-centred planning.

Record keeping

This section will help provide the underpinning knowledge needed for S/NVQ Care Level 2 Unit CU5, 'Receive, transmit, store and retrieve information'.

Whatever your job, you will probably be keeping a record of what you do. You may, for example, write notes each time you make a home care visit and file those notes in a binder kept in the service user's home. If you work in a residential home, then you might write notes in an incident book, or a handover book, or something even more formal, such as an accident book. Records play a very important part in keeping someone's care plan up to date; what you write from day to day (routine as it sometimes sounds) can tell you, and others, a great deal about how well any service is meeting someone's needs. It's also a good idea to look back over your records if you are asked to take part in any kind of review meeting; that should help you feel more confident in planning what you want to say.

Here are some pointers that should help you write the sort of records that will both benefit the people you work with, and meet what's required by the Data Protection Act 1998. Good records should:

- be accurate;
- be up-to-date;
- be reasonably brief;
- be respectful to the service user concerned (a good rule of thumb is 'would I like this written about me?');
- take note of the service user's opinions (but check whether you've got those opinions right before you put them on to paper – what you write stands out, and can often feel more offensive than anything you might have said);
- avoid abbreviations, slang or 'jargon' words that would be hard for others to understand – many of the records you keep are the property of your employer, and may need to be checked by them from time to time;
- separate fact from opinion – for example, 'Alice is very grumpy today' might be a statement of fact, but besides being disrespectful to Alice it doesn't tell us why she is feeling grumpy. 'Alice is very worried about the district nurse's visit tomorrow' is not only respectful to Alice but would also trigger a useful line of discussion if you came to discuss that record with your manager or supervisor, or to use it in a case review;
- always be stored somewhere safe, and/or protected by some form of password if they are saved on your own computer (PC). Many of your records will contain the sort of sensitive information that needs to be kept confidential. As a general rule, records should be shared only with those who need to see them. If you're typing records on to a PC, then make sure no one else can see your screen (and that applies to family members too).

Most records are also a form of public document. They're sometimes the best type of evidence there is that an agency is doing its job properly (ie, what it agreed, or was contracted, to do as part of someone's care plan). In that sense, good records are:

- your own record of good practice;
- a way of telling colleagues what they need to know (like the handover book);
- a way of telling your employer that you're doing a good job;
- a way of telling the world at large that your employer does things properly – this is one way in which employers are held to account for the money they are spending, and the quality of their services;
- a record of someone's life, what they've experienced, and how they've experienced it. This can be very important for people who have lived some time in residential homes; there may be no other way of knowing what has happened to them over the years;
- a way of recording concerns about someone, and what action was taken to meet those concerns.

ACTIVITY 10

Keeping good records

- **How do you think your own records could be improved? Write a sentence or two below.**

Reviewing the care plan

This section will help S/NVQ candidates supply the underpinning knowledge they need for Care Level 2 Units CU10, 'Contribute to the effectiveness of work teams', W2, 'Contribute to the ongoing support of clients and others significant to them', and W3, 'Support individuals experiencing a change in their care requirements and provision'.

Care plans should always be reviewed (they have little long-term value if they don't keep in touch with the service user's progress). Sadly, there are some local authorities that find it very difficult to keep up with the numbers of reviews they need to make (just as there are some service users whose situation changes so rapidly that any review would be quickly out of date). For many older people, reviews will be triggered by an important change in their circumstances, such as an admission to hospital. The strong probability is that at some time you will be invited to join a review meeting.

What part do I play in the review meeting?

It's certainly not a silent part. You may be worried about speaking out in front of strangers, especially when some of them have imposing titles or strange-sounding responsibilities. A good chairperson will be sensitive to these feelings, and will try to bring you into the meeting, even if you are a little hesitant to speak.

These are sometimes fairly formal meetings, where everyone is invited to speak in turn, so it may not be wise to butt in on someone else's contribution too often (even if you don't agree with what they've said). Speak with passion if you wish (there's nothing wrong in speaking up for service users), but try not to make your criticisms too personal. Save any critical comments for someone's actions, not their personality; changing who we are is rather harder than changing what we do.

One of the strengths that care workers or voluntary carers bring to any review is that they often know the person whose care is being reviewed better than many others in the room. Good reviews should always include the service user, though they may be excluded for part of the meeting. If you find yourself having to speak for someone, or to help them put something into their own words, find time to rehearse what you're both going to say before the meeting. That way, you'll each feel more confident about your 'presentation' (and there won't be recriminations afterwards). If, for example, you're asked to pass an opinion on the service user's ability to do things for themselves, then try to put what you say in a way that person would find acceptable – that way you'll feel more comfortable, and more confident about making other contributions to the meeting. There's no doubt that care workers will be asked to take increasing note of what residents say about their quality of care, so you could play an important part in helping older people to be more actively involved in commissioning (or reviewing) their own care packages.

Remember that there cannot legally be a change in the levels of service someone receives unless their circumstances have been reviewed. A service cannot be withdrawn from older or disabled people without first considering their needs and preferences.

ACTIVITY 11

Review meetings

- Think of a review meeting you might have attended/could attend in future. How did you/might you feel before and after that review? Jot down a sentence or two.

Do care planning procedures apply if I don't work for a local authority?

Yes, providing you care for someone whose services are being paid in part by a local authority, or in full by the NHS, since that means they must have had a social services community care assessment, or an NHS continuing care assessment. The same applies if local authorities arrange for someone to be admitted to a residential care home, even if the authority has no financial responsibility for that person. If the person you work for is paying for their own care, then whilst they still have every right to request a community care assessment (or re-assessment), their existing level of service will not necessarily be reviewed. Good practice suggests that anyone receiving a service, however they pay for it, should have their needs (as well as the quality of the service they receive) reviewed from time to time. But, as you saw in 'Working with people who pay for their own care' (page 2), people who pay for their own services are not necessarily in touch with other parts of the welfare system. This puts a special responsibility on their care workers to monitor any change of circumstance and to report back, for example, to their line manager or to one of the other caring agencies, if they think the person they are caring for needs additional support.

Contracts and service specifications

If you work for an agency in the independent or voluntary sectors (see pages xii and xiii), then the likelihood is your employer holds some form of 'contract' to provide a service for older people on behalf of the local authority or the NHS. As you saw in 'The public, state or "statutory" sector' (page xiv), the United Kingdom has a 'mixed economy of care', that is, care is provided by a mixture of 'for-profit' and 'not-for-profit' agencies. It may be that your own contract of employment is fixed to whatever contract(s) your employer currently holds; many carers are employed for short or 'fixed' terms, because the money that pays their salary is guaranteed only for the length of a particular contract(s).

Like anyone else who uses the 'market', local authorities or other bodies purchasing services for older people will want to buy services that meet their requirements for quality and standards at a price they can afford to pay (they must, after all, be able to show local voters, and central government, they are getting the best value for any public money they spend). The problems come (and this is where the way the contracts are priced is not necessarily good news for older service users) when purchasers decide they can get better value from another 'provider', or providers decide they can no longer supply that service at the price being offered. It may be that older people get a better service when suppliers change; it may also be that they lose carers they know and trust, and have to adjust to new faces and new ways of doing things.

Some care agencies have tried to develop a longer-term relationship with local purchasers. These agencies have become 'preferred providers', that is, they have agreed to work to a price and specification the purchaser requires, in return, perhaps, for a guaranteed amount of business each year. One problem with these block contracts (for service users, and often for staff) is that the price agreed may be driven down to a point where it is difficult to provide the highest standards of service.

'Spot' contracts are often the reverse of longer-term contracts; the 'spot' purchase covers one-off or exceptional purchases (eg, buying additional care hours for someone with special needs who wants help over and above the care already purchased for them as part of a longer-term contract). Spot contracts should never be used as a long-term alternative to block contracts.

Any contract will specify the standard of service required from whomever holds it. Some contracts require the providing agency to have procedures in place that could be additional, say, to the registration standards for care homes (eg, an equal opportunities policy, health and safety policies, or policies for the prevention of elder abuse). National standards for home care agencies will shortly be in force.

ACTIVITY 12

Contracts

- **Can you think of any way in which a contract your agency holds affects your day-to-day work with service users? Make some notes overleaf or on the blank pages at the back of this book.**

Making a good referral

S/NVQ candidates may find this section helps provide the underpinning knowledge for Care Level 2 Unit W8, 'Enable individuals to maintain contacts in potentially isolating situations'.

Making a 'referral' is asking for help on someone else's behalf. A good referral needs to be:

- **accurate** – so that all names, addresses etc are correct;
- **appropriate** – because it's gone to the right person or agency (which is what this book is all about)
- **acceptable** – except in emergencies, the older person being referred must know who they are being referred to, and what you are going to say about them; it's not acceptable to refer anyone without their consent.

Paying for services

As you saw in the Introduction, many services in the welfare state are 'means-tested', that is, most service users pay all or part of the cost of any service they receive, depending on their income or other assets (such as savings or property) and the range of charges set for that service. The charges made for home care services are not 'uniform'; that is, they vary from one part of the country to another, or even from borough to borough. The Audit Commission has criticised this practice (*Charging with Care*, 2000), and the government is currently consulting with local authorities about fairer ways to make these charges.

Broadly speaking, if the care an older person receives comes from the local authority (or from one of the agencies which that authority has contracted to work on its behalf), then the person concerned will have to pay for their care according to their means (or 'ability to pay'), unless of course they opt not to disclose their financial circumstances and to pay the full cost for any services they need. If an older person's care comes from the NHS, then because they have a medical or nursing need, no charge will be made for their services, since care in the NHS is 'free at the point of delivery'.

Applying the principles of ability to pay to packages of care that local authorities provide or arrange means that:

- help is given to those who cannot afford to pay (though only 6 per cent of social services departments provide a home care service free of charge to those on the very lowest incomes, NHS Plan 2000);
- the amount charged should not leave someone with less than the basic rate of Income Support to live on;
- service charges are reasonable, and take note of someone's outgoings, like the added costs involved for people with disabilities.

What these principles will mean for you in practice is that:

- you need to know – or, better still, be able to get reliable advice about – the sorts of welfare benefits that help service users 'maximise their income from all legitimate sources';
- you may need to help service users make 'informed choices about how they allocate their regular expenditure' (Meteyard, 1994).

Chapter 2 has a section on welfare benefits (pages 64–72). At this stage, you may find it helpful to know that Age Concern provides a free telephone service (the 'Age Concern Information Line') to members of the public with enquiries about income and money, legal issues, health and community care, housing, and leisure and education. The freephone number (0800 00 99 66) is available from 7.00am to 7.00pm, seven days a week and gives access to a comprehensive range of factsheets on these subjects. There may also be a local Age Concern advice line listed in your telephone directory under 'Age Concern Advice Service'. Citizens Advice Bureaux are another source of informed welfare rights advice; you could go to the Benefits Agency itself (see page 105); and many social services departments have their own welfare rights advisers (sometimes linked to a benefits 'hotline'). Some social services departments also publish a guide to their charging policies.

By and large, you should avoid giving advice on such areas of personal finance as houses, estates, pensions, savings and investments. Far too many older people are reluctant to ask for advice, and go without the help to which they are properly entitled. Personal finance is a complex area, so that advice on these issues needs to come from people who are qualified to give it. Meddle and get things wrong, and you could make it difficult for an older person to ask for advice again. 'The principle here is no advice is better than poor advice' (Meteyard, 1994).

If you are working in a care home, you may know residents who, in order to pay for their care, have sold property they had hoped would be an inheritance for members of their family. The Royal Commission on Long Term Care was set up to report on this and other problems involved in funding the long-term care of older people. The Commission recommended that personal care should be paid from general taxation, but that other living costs, such as food or board, should be 'subject to payment according to means' (*With Respect to Old Age*, 1999). The government did not accept these recommendations, though they did accept that nursing care should be free to care and nursing home residents from October 2001 (a rather thorny issue, since nursing care and social care are sometimes hard to separate); that residents could keep a little more of their capital before becoming liable for care home fees; and that new residents should not be forced to dispose of any property they own before they have lived in the home for three months (NHS Plan 2000).

Now, as many of you will know, many older people are worried or angered about the amounts they pay for care, either care in their own homes, or care in residential homes. It's very important that the advice older people receive about financial matters is correct and up-to-date. If you are asked for such advice, then check out what you say before risking a mistake. The Age Concern Welfare Rights Service (see page 65) will be able to help you (as will other welfare rights services, or the Citizens Advice Bureau).

2 The roles of care team members

If you look back to the beginning of this book, you'll see from the Introduction how important it is that carers 'feel part of the caring "team", whether or not they have "professional" qualifications'. There are two good reasons why care workers should feel they are respected members of that team:

- they usually spend far more time with the older person than other team members (making them likely to know *what is important to that person*, and *who is important to them*);
- they are particularly well placed to monitor, or keep in touch with, any changes in the older person's circumstances.

Because they know the older person so well, care workers will often feel the need to speak on that person's behalf, especially, as you've already seen, when that person comes into contact with other members of the caring team, such as social workers, nurses and doctors. Most of this chapter has been designed to help you understand the roles and responsibilities of care team members; the more you understand about the work of colleague team members, the more you will be able to use their help on behalf of someone you care for. That means speaking up for them, and often speaking up for yourself as well (though, as you saw in Chapter 1, speaking up for someone is not quite the same thing as being their 'spokesperson', something referred to again on the next page).

To help you make the best possible job of speaking up for older people whenever the need arises, this chapter starts with a section on advocacy *(though all these sections will help S/NVQ candidates working on Care Level 2 Units W8, 'Enable individuals to maintain contacts in potentially isolating situations', and Z8, 'Support individuals when they are distressed').*

Advocacy

Do older people need advocates?

It's known from research studies (like Barner et al, 1982) that older people need more help in referring themselves to welfare services than any other group in the population: they need someone to help make that referral for them (remember what you wrote about 'officialdom' in Activity 6). There's also a sense in which many older people are particularly dependent on welfare services: they may be very frail, for example, and need a great deal of help with just maintaining their day-to-day lives. It's very easy to overlook someone's needs in this situation, not because we are being deliberately unkind, but because *our* ways of doing things gradually come to take the place of *their* ways of doing things. Older people can feel themselves losing control just as soon as they start to depend on other people to do things they once did for themselves. Of course, not every older person will put their feelings into quite those words, but next time you're tempted to see someone as a 'whinger' or grumbler, think what it's like, for example, to get your breakfast not when you want it, but when your home carer struggles in out of a traffic jam to get it for you.

It's in situations like these that older people need someone to help them take back a little of the power they may have lost. Think about the following quotation. It comes from a study by the Social Care Practice Centre at Warwick University. A group of care home residents had told researchers at the University how much they disliked weekly baths by rota, 'rules' they couldn't do anything to influence, and the feeling they were 'different' from everyone else. This is what the University concluded: 'for some older people there is an overwhelming sense of powerlessness and lack of control with individuality and personal preferences sacrificed' (*Care Weekly*, 5 June 1992). These were people who needed to feel more 'empowered'.

ACTIVITY 13

Empowerment

- **In your experience, how do older people become 'disempowered'? Write a sentence or two below.**

Should I always act as someone's advocate?

No. There may be times when you're too close to the older person concerned to separate what you want to say from what they want to say. There will also be times when it's you who are part of the problem (eg, when there's something the older person wants you to do differently, but they can't quite find a way to put that request into words). Being employed as an older person's care worker may be at odds with being their 'advocate'. If that person has a problem with the standard of care they receive, you may feel you have to defend your own position. You may also feel a loyalty to your employer that may put you in a difficult position (so that you're pulled in two directions at once).

There are other times when speaking out may not achieve all you'd hoped for. Finding the right person to act on your concerns isn't quite as easy as it sounds. Other members of the caring team may fail to act on what you've said to them because they don't have authority to take appropriate action. If you're worried about what to say, and when to say it, then talk to your line manager, or trade union representative, or encourage the older person to make a complaint (since every complaint must be properly investigated). It may also be that the older person needs help of a very technical nature (eg, handling an appeal against a decision to limit their welfare benefits); in that case, the wiser course of action might be for you to seek help from a more experienced colleague.

An option in any situation where you cannot advocate yourself is to use someone else as an 'independent advocate'. For example, where an older person has some form of disability, the Disabled Persons Act 1986 makes it possible for an independent advocate to be given whatever information a local authority would give the disabled person themselves. Advocates also have a right to talk to anyone in private.

Carers' groups will also advocate on behalf of their members. Someone acting as an independent advocate to an older or disabled person you care for may approach you directly. If you find yourself in this position, then remember that the advocate's first loyalty is to the person they are speaking for. If they are critical of something you have done, the likelihood is that their criticism is not directed at you personally (though it may sound that way) so much as being directed through you to the agency that employs you, or the procedures that agency wants you to use.

Effective advocacy in practice

You'll have seen from Chapter 1 that, whatever the advantages of independent advocacy, assessments and case reviews give you the opportunity (if not an open invitation) to speak on behalf of older people in your care. Advocates are not there to represent their own point of view (or even, like spokespeople, to 'represent' a set of views that others share). Advocates are there to give someone else a voice that might not otherwise be heard. There are four principles of effective advocacy below; you'll see they are consistent with much of what you've worked on in Chapter 1:

- speaking up for or acting on behalf of yourself or another person;
- making sure a person's voice is heard;
- making sure a person's needs are met;
- making sure a person knows their rights and has the information to make informed choices and get the benefits and services they are entitled to.

ACTIVITY 14

Advocacy in practice

- Think back to a meeting where you had to (or would have liked to) speak up for someone whose voice wouldn't otherwise be heard. Which principles applied to what you said or would have liked to say? Make a brief note showing how the principles fitted what you said. Use the space below, or preferably the blank pages at the back of this book. *S/NVQ candidates should find these notes are useful 'knowledge evidence' for Units CL1, 'Promote effective communication and relationships', and CL2, 'Promote communication with individuals where there are communication differences'.*

The Carers' National Strategy and Carers' Charters

Many paid and, particularly, unpaid carers put the needs of the people they care for before their own (which is why they have a right to have their own needs considered by any 'professional' caring team). As Prime Minister Tony Blair wrote in 1999, 'Carers devote large parts of their own lives to the lives of others – not as part of a job, but voluntarily. And often in addition to working themselves'. Voluntary caring is sometimes seen as the cement that holds many communities together; it's a 'vital part of the fabric and character of Britain' (*Caring about Carers*, 1999). Existing services would collapse without the care so many older people receive from friends and family. Yet here are some figures that might surprise you:

- One out of every eight people in Britain gives care to somebody – that's close to 6 million people.
- Women are more likely to care voluntarily than men, though there are proportionately more men aged 65 and over than women caring for a disabled partner (General Household Survey, 1992).
- Three-fifths of people who care voluntarily are looking after someone with a disability.
- 855,000 voluntary carers provide care for more than 50 hours each week.
- Three-fifths of all voluntary carers *receive no regular visitor support services at all.*
- Adult children and their parents exchange a great deal of help in everyday tasks, like giving lifts in cars, shopping, domestic chores, paperwork, and household maintenance (*Social Trends*, 2001).

ACTIVITY 15

Carers' isolation

- **Make a note below of anyone in your immediate neighbourhood you think of as a voluntary carer (including yourself if appropriate). How many of those people are in regular contact with the caring services?**

To help all organisations involved with caring to focus 'not just on the client, patient, or user', but also on their carer(s), the government introduced a 'national strategy for carers'. There are three elements to that strategy:

1 Information including a new charter on what people can expect from long-term care services; an extension of the NHS Direct telephone helpline to include information specifically for carers; and more government information for carers 'posted' on the Internet (see http://www.gov.uk).
2 Support for carers to be involved in the planning and provision of services.
3 Care with an emphasis on carers' rights to have their own health needs met; new powers for local authorities to provide services for carers, as well as those being cared for; and extra money specifically to services that help carers to take a break.

At local level, both carers themselves and agencies concerned about them have been encouraged to commit themselves to the principles of a Carer's Charter (and to develop, or help develop, action plans that put those principles into practice). The seven principles below, for example, are taken from the *Charter for Carers in Suffolk* (1999):

- Carers should have *recognition*.
- Carers should have *choice*.
- Carers should have *information*.
- Carers should be provided with appropriate *practical help*.
- The financial *cost of caring* should be *minimised*.
- *Services* and information should be *co-ordinated* within and across agencies in order to best meet the needs of carers.
- Carers should be *involved* in planning and monitoring the services they receive.

ACTIVITY 16

The Carer's Charter

- **Look out a copy of the Carer's Charter for the area where you live or work. Any carers' association will probably have a copy they can send you, or you can ask if your line manager**

has a copy. Check to see whether any organisations you are associated with, or work for, are committed to implementing the Charter (organisations 'adopting' the Charter will be named in the leaflet). If you find your organisation has not adopted the Charter, then ask an appropriate person if they can explain that decision to you.

Working with carers (ie, paid carers working with unpaid carers)

You may well be working for an agency that's taken part in designing (and is now committed to implementing) a local Carer's Charter. You may also be helping to provide a short-break service funded from the Carer's or Promoting Independence Grants (ie, one of the 'care' components in the Carers' National Strategy, above). A stronger probability still is that you are working with carers, ie, the relatives, friends and neighbours of older people you, as paid carers, care for too. Here are some pointers that will help you develop and maintain these very important relationships. *S/NVQ candidates will find this useful knowledge evidence for Care Level 2 Units CL1, 'Promote effective communication and relationships', and W8, 'Enable individuals to maintain contacts in potentially isolating situations'.*

The Carers (Recognition and Services) Act 1995, and the Carers and Disabled Children Act 2000 give voluntary carers a legal right to have their needs assessed (whether or not the person they care for has had their needs assessed, and even if that person has refused an assessment: Carers and Disabled Children Act 2000, Summary 2001). As you may know from your own experience, carers' needs are all too easily submerged by the needs of those they care for. It's not that carers' needs have been completely invisible up to now (friends and family may have been very worried about them, for example, as might other professional carers): it's just that services have never been geared to seeing carers as 'co-clients' (Banks, 1998), ie, as service users in their own right, or to building partnerships between paid and unpaid carers. Sharing is what partnerships are all about. Your job as a care worker is to 'share the care' of someone who may be very precious to others caring for them. What this means in practice is that:

1 There will be times when the right and proper thing for you to do is to care for the carer too (and if that isn't in the care plan you're working to, then you may have to 'speak up' on that carer's behalf); and
2 You need to work out what you're going to do for the older person being cared for *in consultation* with their friends and family.

Voluntary carers also need the opportunity to make choices. They need to choose whether or not they continue, or take on, the caring role. Try to help them make such choices by using the techniques set out in 'Making choices and direct payments' (page 3). Carers often have great difficulty juggling the demands of their working lives, their personal lives, and their caring lives. You should never assume that anyone wants, or is able, to take on additional caring responsibilities, whatever their cultural background. This (in part) is what the government means by giving carers 'the freedom to have a life of their own' (*Caring about Carers*, 1999).

If you work in a residential home, you may know that many of the people who previously cared for a resident still want to feel involved in that person's life, even though they have had to move into residential care. Though it's much harder to share someone's care in these circumstances, the home's routines mustn't become an excuse for not involving friends and family who wish to stay in touch with the care of a loved one (and some homes have found ingenious ways of helping carers play a part in the care of someone they once looked after). Being in residential care can become a very lonely experience; sadly, we sometimes make it harder for caring relationships to continue once someone moves to a home by putting obstacles in the previous carer's way (eg, making it difficult for residents to entertain their friends in private or to offer them a cup of tea). Before you fall for the old chestnut that relatives don't visit because they are eaten up with guilt about 'putting someone away', look round at how welcome your home makes visitors feel when they do call.

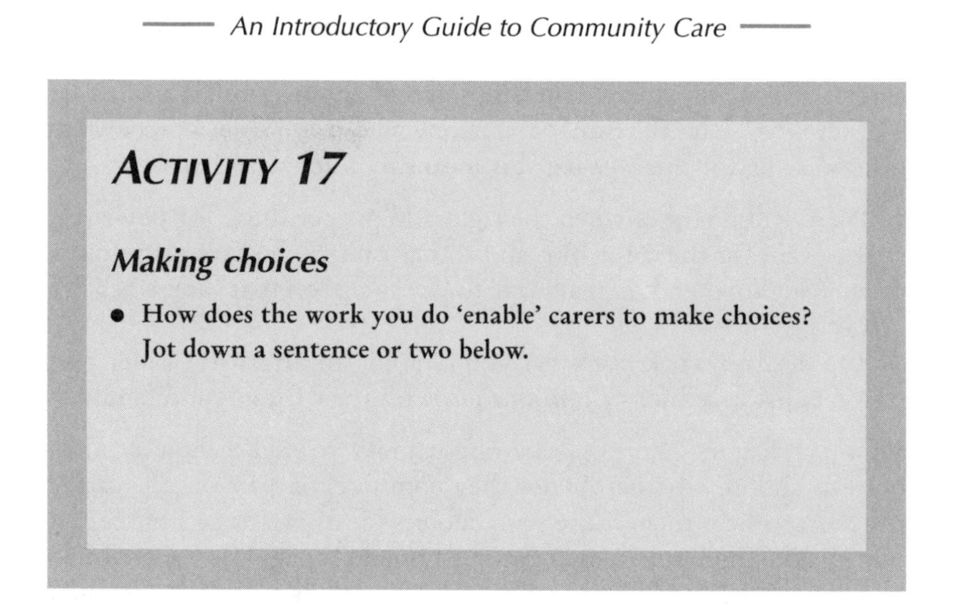

ACTIVITY 17

Making choices

- How does the work you do 'enable' carers to make choices? Jot down a sentence or two below.

Social work and social services/social work departments

This is where you'll start to learn about other roles and responsibilities in the 'caring team'.

Social services are pretty big business. Nationally, 'social services deal with over 1.5 million people and their families every year, employing directly or indirectly some one million care staff. Most people, or their friends and relatives, will have contact with social services during some part of their lives' (*So what do social workers do?* 1999).

Different arrangements for different parts of the country

As you saw in the Introduction, there are different arrangements for the provision of social services in different parts of the country. England and Wales have social services departments; Scotland has social work departments; and Northern Ireland has health and social services boards. Outside Northern Ireland, every department is part of a local authority. In English rural areas, many social services departments are part of the local county council (not the district councils). Elsewhere, social services and social work departments are parts of a 'unitary' authority (combining social services, education, *and* housing services), or they are parts of metropolitan district councils or London Boroughs (both of which also have housing responsibilities, unlike county councils, which do not).

ACTIVITY 18

Finding the right department

- **Find out the full name of your local social services/social work department, including the local council that department is part of. Write down your answer below.**

A key distinction

There is an important distinction between field staff in social service departments and staff who work in residential and day services (as you probably do yourself). 'Field' staff include most social workers, and others, such as social work 'assistants' and occupational therapists, who visit service users at home; are not generally expected to work shifts; and usually have an office they are 'based' at (see below). Residential and day service staff will work in homes for older people, at day centres (though many day services for older people are provided by voluntary organisations) and in the home care service. Though they use by far the larger part of social service budgets, residential and day services have always been something of a 'poor relation' by comparison with fieldwork services; no more than 20 per cent of the staff in these services hold any form of professional qualification, for example, and few staff in senior management posts have used residential and day service jobs as a stepping stone to promotion. From October 2001, the General Social Care Council (GSCC) for England will be responsible for setting codes of conduct and practice for social care workers and their employers (in the same way that nurses, for instance, have codes of conduct); for 'registering' the social care workforce (a task that will take some time to complete, given so few of the social care workforce hold relevant qualifications); and regulating professional social work education (mainly for social workers). There are also targets set for increasing the numbers of social care staff holding relevant qualifications. As part of the National Training Strategy for England, 50 per cent of all residential care staff in adult services will be expected to have an appropriate National Vocational Qualification (NVQ) by 2005 (*Modernising the Social Care Workforce*, TOPSS, 2000).

Specialist 'teams'

Social services are generally organised into specialist 'teams' or sections; that is, the team specialises in working with the kinds of people that section serves. Most community care services for older people will be part of an 'adult', as distinct from a children's, service; other parts of the same department will be responsible for services to children, young people and their families, people with mental health problems, and people with disabilities (including learning disabilities). In Scotland, social work departments also provide a service to the courts, and to children's hearings or panels, that elsewhere in the country is the responsibility of the probation services (the Scottish legal system makes very different arrangements for children and young people in any kind of difficulty). Some field staff work in 'multi-disciplinary' teams (especially in mental health and learning disability services); their fellow team members are usually community psychiatric nurses.

Many social services departments are housed in some form of council buildings, though some of their staff are based in GP surgeries, some use high street shop fronts, or offices in residential homes or day centres, and some are beginning to be 'based' in their own homes (with 'caller points' elsewhere for people wanting to visit them). Some departments share 'one-stop shops' with staff from the local housing department and/or other welfare agencies (see 'Hospital and hospice social workers' below). Some departments have a single telephone number for all their enquiries; you can find this, and other telephone numbers, under 'Social Services' in the business section of your local telephone directory.

As you may have experienced yourself, many social services departments have re-organised their local boundaries in line with the boundaries used by primary care groups in the health service (see page 50). This should make it easier for health and social services staff to build good working relationships with each other.

Hospital and hospice social workers

For the most part, all but the smallest cottage or GP hospitals will generally have social service staff based at the hospital, and even the smaller hospitals have social workers who visit them on a regular basis. Social workers play an important part in patient care by addressing the sorts of emotional, family, or practical problems that sometimes slow someone's recovery or delay their discharge from hospital. In psychiatric hospitals and hospitals for people with learning disabilities, social workers will link with patients and their carers, sometimes helping prepare and provide that person with 'care in the community' (as distinct from care in hospital, not quite the same, for instance, as providing community care for someone living in their own home). Hospital social workers also help prepare the sorts of community care assessments that pave the way for many older people to leave hospital with an appropriate care plan. Hospice social workers will often help to link the medical team to patients and their families, helping prepare the family for bereavement, and supporting them once their loved one has died.

Hospital-based social workers are generally employed by local authorities, and not by hospital trusts (except in Northern Ireland, where health and social services are combined). Many hospice social workers are employed by the hospice itself (since hospices are often voluntary organisations, supported by, but not a part of, the NHS). Hospital social workers are often attached to particular wards or sections of the hospital, eg, oncology (cancer), renal or paediatric (children's) units.

Social services responsibilities for community care

These sound rather formal, but each of the words in *italics* should take your mind back to something you've read earlier in this book:

- Making *information* accessible to potential customers and carers on the types of services available, the criteria for providing services, the assessment and complaints procedures and the standards by which those procedures will be measured.
- *Assessing* community care needs, negotiated and agreed with other agencies.
- *Communicating* the outcome of assessments to customers, carers and other parties to the process.
- *Reviewing* individual care needs at regular intervals.
- Feeding back information about community care needs into the service *planning* system.

(Suffolk Health and Social Services, 1997)

- Along with setting *eligibility criteria* for services they provide or arrange.

Social workers and social work 'assistants'

What do they do?

One of the people you are likely to meet in any case review will be a social worker. Here are some of the tasks that any social worker is likely to carry out:

Assessment, as, for example, in preparing a community care assessment. Assessment has become a very important activity for social workers, especially those involved in work with older people. The sorts of care needs social workers recognise when they carry out community care assessments add up to the services a social services department needs to purchase. Assessment can be broken down into six steps:

- noting the problem;
- forming an impression;
- collecting additional information where needed;

- thinking out the nature of the problem;
- deciding what action to take;
- keeping everyone aware of whatever decisions are made.

Providing services and advice is another important social work activity. As you saw earlier on, the outcome of any assessment is often a care plan. The care plan will specify which services an older person requires. Welfare benefits advice could be a significant part of that plan.

Monitoring or surveillance (though not the kind of surveillance you see in TV crime dramas) is what reviews are all about. It's keeping in touch with people whose needs are likely to change. Monitoring becomes a very important activity for some groups of vulnerable people. If someone is at serious risk of harming themselves or others, then social workers will sometimes have the power to intervene, and move that person somewhere safe, such as a residential home or a hospital.

Mediating is putting people in touch with voluntary groups, with activities in their local neighbourhood, or with any other activity or service written into someone's care plan. The skill of mediating is building a bridge between the service user and the new service they are going to use (ie, giving information, calming anxieties and 'speaking up' for what the service user needs).

Counselling involves discussions with the service user, or their family and friends, where the aim, taking very careful note of everyone's feelings, is to 'help that person change or adapt some aspect of their life or relationships' (*Social Workers: Their Role and Tasks*, NISW, 1982). The use of counselling skills is often part of other tasks the social worker carries out. Think, for example, of the counselling skills that may be required when older people come to making difficult decisions about their future living arrangements, especially when family relationships are strained or complicated.

Activity 19

Assessment stages

- Think of any assessment that you've observed, or been part of. How many stages could you pick out in the way the assessment was put together? At what stage(s) is consultation with service users important? Use the space below to jot down your answers.

What does specialisation mean?

If social workers 'specialise' in work with one group of service users, say older people, they are unlikely to work with other groups of service users too (ie, specialists in work with older people will not be asked to include children and young people on their workload). When social services departments first came into being, in 1971, many social workers were urged to work 'across the board' with all groups of service users, but the introduction of the NHS and Community Care Act 1990, with its emphasis on care management, gave a strong spur to specialisation.

What is the difference between social workers and social work assistants?

Social workers almost always hold a professional qualification (a requirement under the Care Standards Act 2001): social work 'assistants' (whom you may know as community care practitioners, social services officers, or care co-ordinators) will probably not be qualified. As a somewhat rough-and-ready way of separating what social workers and social work assistants do, you can think of social workers, because of their qualifications, being given work that is rather more complicated than the work done by social work assistants. Social workers will be used, for example, where there is a strong element of risk to the service user involved; where relationships between the service user and their friends or family are particularly fraught or difficult; where the service user's mental health is particularly frail; or where their needs seem especially complex. Social work assistants will be used where the likely 'care package' following assessment looks to be fairly straightforward, such as providing a meals service, and home care (though as always with fine judgements of this sort, what looks straightforward often turns out to be unexpectedly complicated). Most social workers and social work assistants are likely to be women.

Will I meet other social service specialists?

Yes, possibly. Here are some other groups of social services staff involved in the care of older people:

Social workers for the blind or deaf work with people who are newly blind or deaf, will almost always be known to members of the blind or deaf 'community', will help with mobility training for people who are blind, or advise on aids for people who are blind or deaf. Social workers for the deaf will sometimes 'interpret' for people who normally 'sign', though some departments use interpreters trained to a high standard in the use of British Sign Language (BSL).

Approved social workers are the only group of social workers with the training and the legal authority to admit someone to a psychiatric hospital compulsorily (ie, whether or not that person agrees to be admitted). This is sometimes called admitting someone 'on section' (because the legal powers used come under a 'Section' of the Mental Health Act 1983). It may be that an older person in your care is so much at risk of harming themselves or others that they need compulsory admission to hospital (though these powers are rarely used for people who are mentally confused).

Social workers (learning disability) may be involved in the care of an older person who also has a learning disability, especially when that person's care plan is reviewed, or if they need additional services.

Occupational therapists, and **'OT aids' occupational therapists**, or **'OTs'** (all of whom are professionally qualified) are employed in both social services and the health service. Both health and social service OTs will visit service users in their own homes, where they often advise on the sorts of aids and adaptations that will help an older person retain their mobility or independence. They also advise on 'specialist housing needs', such as fitting a stair lift or adding a downstairs bathroom or toilet. Unfortunately, many local authorities find it hard to recruit OTs, and there is often a lengthy waiting list for social service OT visits. OT assistants, who may be training as OTs, will sometimes fit the simpler aids, such as bath rails or toilet seats. A charge may be made for aids and equipment recommended by social services OTs (but not for the same equipment recommended by health service OTs). Some social service departments still provide a craft teaching service, which might be used, for example, by residents in care homes.

ACTIVITY 20

Finding the right kinds of help

- **Could any people you are working with benefit from social services help they don't seem to be receiving? Make a note of what you think such people need, and show it to your line manager or supervisor.**

Social service management

Social services departments are required by law to have a Director of Social Services ('Director of Social Work' in Scotland), though many of the newer local authorities have combined their social service and housing 'directorates'. Directors in England, Wales and Scotland report to an elected committee of local councillors. Though we know that local voters often stay away from the polls, and that the Cabinet-style committees used by many local authorities can be very powerful, a significant difference between health and social services is that whilst health service managers must consult with local people, social service policies can be challenged by local voters through the ballot box, ie, they can vote out the councillors controlling social services committees every time there is a local election. Devolution also means that decisions on welfare services in Scotland and Wales (and ultimately in Northern Ireland) can be challenged through elections to the Scottish Parliament and the Welsh and Northern Irish Assemblies.

Age discrimination in health and social care

Why do we need to think about age discrimination? Well, principally because many people are very concerned about it, so much so that the government is committed to eradicating age-related discrimination in health and social services as part of the National Service Framework for Older People (2001), and Age Concern England is currently campaigning to end 'discrimination against older people – by law' (*Age Concern's priorities for the next parliament*, 2001).

So what do we mean by age discrimination? This is how the King's Fund describes it: 'Age discrimination results from ageism which is a form of prejudice. Despite the fact that the majority of older people describe themselves as being in good health (less than one per cent of the older population is in hospital at any one time), older people tend to be stereotyped as a ... group characterised by passivity, failing mental health, and dependency' (*Age discrimination in health and social care*, 2000).

What does this mean in practice? It means that older people tend to be offered services that younger people might not want to rely on themselves. The excuse we make, of course, and it's less an excuse than an example of just how prejudiced we can be, is that older people, especially very old people, have 'had a good innings', so when it comes to dividing out funds that might improve existing resources a larger share goes to services for younger people. Here are some examples of how such prejudice works. Both health and social services staff who work with older people tend to be less well qualified than staff who work with other user groups (though the National Training Strategy sets targets to increase the numbers of care workers holding NVQs: *Modernising the Social Care Workforce*, TOPSS, 2000). Care workers are not well paid. The speedy provision of aids and equipment (so important for preserving the dignity and independence of older people) has not been given the priority it deserves. In the health service, clinical trials and medical research have tended to exclude older people, and although this is changing, the risk is that older people develop complications through drug interactions that have not been tested on younger people. GPs can also be reluctant to provide annual health checks for people over 75, missing an opportunity to identify potential health problems, and to give advice on healthy living. 'Older people from black and minority ethnic groups often face double discrimination from health' or social care 'services that are neither culturally competent nor well-suited to supporting older people's health' (*King's Fund News*, 2000). All NHS Departments must assess their policies for treatment of the elderly by October 2001 to ensure that no decisions are made on the basis of age alone (ANANOVA, 2001).

Community health services

This part of Chapter 2 begins by looking very briefly at how community health services are organised. The remainder of this rather long section describes the sorts of community health services older people in your care are likely to use. By giving you a better understanding of the help your health service colleagues give older people, we hope you will encourage such people to make the best possible use of those services. Good health care, like any other part of good community care, improves someone's 'quality of life' and helps maintain their independence. At the start of a century when average life expectancies may continue to increase, there really isn't much excuse for dumbing down the health care problems older people experience as 'just old age'.

NHS 'trusts'

You've probably seen your local hospital, for example, described as an 'NHS trust'. You might be employed by a trust, or working alongside, say, district nurses employed by a 'community trust'. There are several kinds of trust (depending on the services they provide), though the likelihood is you'll come into contact with either a hospital trust (usually based on one of the larger 'district general' hospitals), a community trust or a mental health trust. Community trusts provide the sorts of services people use in their own homes, such as district nursing. They sometimes provide hospital services too, though generally for people with mental health problems, or learning disabilities (ie, there isn't a separate mental health trust in that area).

All NHS trusts have a board of directors. Some directors look after the day-to-day management of the trust (these are the 'executive' directors); others (the 'non-executive' directors) are appointed by the local health authority or the Secretary of State because of the experience they bring from other forms of community service. Trusts have a lot more freedom in the way they manage their affairs than, say, the hospital management committees that preceded them. They can also do things that an ordinary business might do, such as borrow money (though within limitations) and decide how much to pay their staff (though, again, within limitations). For the most part, the income any trust receives comes either from health authorities or, in England, from the new primary care groups (PCGs). The functions of health authorities and PCGs are briefly described below.

Health authorities

Health authorities plan, finance and monitor health services for people in the areas they serve, via primary care groups, and primary care trusts (see below). Health authorities probably fund most of the health services provided in your area. They also 'plan, develop, and monitor' services provided by GPs, dentists, retail pharmacists and opticians. Increasingly, they fund and commission community services as a joint venture with social services. 'Building healthy communities' is not something any authority can do single-handedly, and health authorities must 'work in partnership with GPs, NHS trusts, and local authorities, as well as members of the public, voluntary, public and private organisations' (Suffolk Health, 1999).

Primary care groups

Primary care groups (PCGs) are a way of localising the planning or 'commissioning' of English health care services. Health authorities typically cover a relatively large area, like a combination of boroughs, or a shire county; PCGs cover much smaller areas (about 100,000 people). There are approximately 480 PCGs in England (2001), and all GP practices belong to one of them. They replace 'fund-holding' GP practices, where GPs held a budget they could use to purchase services for patients using their practice. PCGs work within the powers and budgets delegated to them by their local health authority. The primary care 'group' is governed by a board that includes up to seven local GPs and nurses, a representative from social services, and at least two 'lay' members, who might, for example, represent a carers' group. Lay members are also expected to make themselves available to local people concerned about the quality or availability of health services in their area (though anyone with complaints about a particular service would be better advised to make a formal complaint to the agency concerned). To an extent, PCGs also restore the freedoms some GPs lost (if they weren't part of a fund-holding practice), for example, to direct patients to a hospital of their choosing. GPs now decide collectively (as part of the PCG) where to fund the services they want to use. By April 2004, all PCGs will be expected to provide some of the services they currently commission; that is, they will become 'primary care trusts' (PCTs).The first of these was set up in autumn 2000. Scotland has primary care trusts rather than primary care groups; Scottish PCTs are responsible for local services to frail elderly people, people with learning disabilities, and people with mental health problems. Scotland also has a system of local health care 'co-operatives', less formal than the English PCGs, but with roughly similar functions. Wales will have local health groups (LHGs), but no health authorities.

Care trusts

The NHS Plan 2000 talks of removing the 'outdated institutional barriers between health and social care that have got in the way of people getting the care they need when they need it.' Too many older people had 'fallen into cracks' between the health and social services (NHS Plan 2000). The Health Act 1999 paved the way for a much closer relationship between health and social services by making it possible for them to employ each other's staff, to pool their budgets, and to provide services jointly. Care trusts will provide for 'even closer integration of health and social services ... by commissioning and taking responsibility for all local health and social care' (NHS Plan 2000).

Now you may think this sounds a little like the primary care trusts you've just read about, and you'd be right. What the government intends to do is build on the development of primary care trusts, and their provision of community services, in areas where health and social services want to follow this particular route to closer integration. These new organisations will be known as care trusts because they have a wider range of functions than primary care trusts, and because their boards will need the sort of membership that represents this new health and social care 'partnership'. Care trusts will be able to commission and deliver primary and community health care as well as social care for older people and other groups of service users (though social services will have to be delivered under delegated authority from the local authority(ies) concerned).

Health Improvement Programmes

Every health authority in the country had to produce its first 'Health Improvement Programme' (HImP) by April 1999 (HImP1). One of the government's priorities is to ensure that everyone has access to the sort of 'quality' health care services that help them live longer, healthier lives, no matter what they earn or which part of the country they live in. Health authorities cannot purchase all the services that help people lead healthier lives. A variety of things affect our health, for example:

- whether we have a job, and what sort of job that is;
- pollution;

- whether we take enough exercise, or whether we smoke;
- the sorts of homes we live in.

Because so many factors go to building healthy communities, HImPs must be drawn up by a 'partnership' of organisations, including the NHS trusts, PCGs, local authorities, voluntary organisations, and 'organisations representing the users of services and their carers'. Current HImPs will concentrate on one of five priorities:

- reducing deaths from heart disease and strokes;
- reducing deaths from cancer;
- improving mental health;
- reducing accidents and injuries;
- reducing health inequalities.

Don't be surprised, therefore, if you see in your local HImP a commitment from local authorities that reads something like: 'the introduction of new cycle routes, 20 mph zones, and other traffic calming measures', since that both reduces accidents (to cyclists and pedestrians) and reduces the risk of death from heart disease and strokes (by encouraging more people to cycle rather than using their cars). Health authorities want you, or any organisation you represent, to contribute to HImPs. To get a copy of the HImP for your area, or to find out more about your contribution to that programme, contact your local health authority; the address and telephone number will be in the phone book. From 2003, HImPs must also include Local Health Improvement Programmes (co-ordinated by PCGs, and their equivalent bodies in Scotland and Wales).

ACTIVITY 21

Quality services

- **You can see that the 'commissioning' of health services is getting much closer to the experience of people who actually**

use those services. That means there will be more people planning those services, and more variation in the services provided from area to area (depending on local needs and preferences). Can you think why 'this Government wants to see a *National* Health Service which offers dependable, high standards of care and treatment everywhere'? (*A First Class Service: Quality in the New NHS*, 1998). What you read about 'inequalities' in the previous section should give you a clue. Write a sentence or two below.

The 'primary care' services

These are services most of us are likely to be familiar with (since they are often based at the local GP surgery). They are also a 'way in' or 'point of access' to other specialist services; GPs, for example, will usually arrange for someone to be admitted to hospital or to see a 'specialist'. Within the general umbrella of primary care services we can include general medical practitioners (or GPs), dentists, pharmacists, opticians, nurses, health visitors, and school nurses, as well as the community health service staff employed by NHS trusts (in community psychiatric services, for instance).

Intermediate care

Intermediate care is a key priority in the National Service Framework for Older People (2001). What is meant by intermediate care is a range of services designed to prevent older people from going into hospital unnecessarily; or to speed up their discharge from hospital and to help them back into leading a normal life at home (*Rehabilitation and intermediate care for older people*, King's Fund, 2000). 'Too many older people are admitted to hospital for the want of community based services that would better meet their needs. Consequently, they are running unnecessary risks of disruption to their social networks, disorientation and hospital acquired infections' (National Service Framework for Older People, Executive Summary, 2001). Here are some examples of the intermediate care facilities that the Department of Health expects health authorities, primary care groups and primary care trusts to have in place by March 2004:

- Rapid response teams, made up of nurses, therapists, care workers, social workers, therapists and GPs working to provide emergency care for people at home and helping to prevent unnecessary hospital admissions.
- Intensive rehabilitation services, to help older patients regain their health and independence after a stroke or major surgery. These will normally be situated in hospitals.
- Recuperation facilities: many patients are not fit enough to go home but do not need hospital care; short-term care in a nursing home or other special accommodation eases the passage for them.
- Arrangements at GP-practice or social-work level to ensure that older people receive a 'one-stop' service: this might mean employing or designating a link or key worker, or basing care managers in GP surgeries.
- Integrated home care teams, so that when people are discharged from hospital they receive the care they need to help them live independently at home.

The NHS Plan provides an extra £900 million to be invested in intermediate care and 'related services' designed to 'promote independence and improve the quality of life for older people' (NHS Plan 2000, Chapter 7).

Rehabilitation services

Rehabilitation is not necessarily the same thing as intermediate care. As you saw above, someone receiving intermediate care might need 'intensive rehabilitation services' to help get them out of hospital, but it's just as likely that someone using rehabilitation services is being helped to stay at home (which is why these services need to be developed at the same time as intermediate care services). Rehabilitation is a relatively short-term but 'active process of building up a person's capacity to live independently' (*Rehabilitation and intermediate care for older people*, 2000). It might, for instance, include 'social rehabilitation', such as helping someone regain a vital self-help skill like preparing meals or making cups of tea, or it might involve something more directly related to health care needs, such as wound care or symptom control. As you can see, the importance of rehabilitation or 're-ablement' (whether or not the work you do is actually given that name) is that it helps the older person regain a skill(s) they have temporarily lost (following a stay in hospital, perhaps, or a crisis at home). Care workers can play an important part in the 'rehabilitation team' (along with doctors, nurses, and therapists), providing they have the right kinds of training and support. Equally, 'if the user (of rehabilitation services) has a carer at home, for example, a spouse or son/daughter, the carer should also be seen as a member of the rehabilitation team, with an important contribution to make' (*Rehabilitation and intermediate care for older people*, 2000). As you can see, there are three 'defining' characteristics of rehabilitation:

- It restores people to a previous state; ie, it gets them back, as far as possible, to where they were before the event which brought about their need for rehabilitation.
- It is purposeful: anyone involved in rehabilitation needs to set some form of goal to measure their progress; unlike convalescence, rehabilitation doesn't come about with the passage of time.
- It is diverse: it involves a variety of service-user needs being met by a broadly based 'rehabilitation team'.

(Nocon and Baldwin, 1998)

General practitioners (or family doctors)

GPs are responsible for providing 24-hour general medical care (though they may use a 'locum' service for out-of-hours calls). GPs play a very important role in ensuring the continuity of someone's care (think, for example, how long you have known your own GP). Each GP practice (though not necessarily the building in which it is housed) is owned by the doctor(s) involved, either singly or in partnership with others. This is why the 'practice' employs some of the staff who work there, such as the receptionists, translators and the practice manager (if there is one). About 60 per cent of what GPs earn comes from 'capitation fees' for each patient registered with them. The rest is made up of fees for minor surgery, family planning advice, and fees for meeting 'targets', such as the numbers of immunisations given by the practice or the numbers of home visits made by individual GPs. Patients can register with any GP they choose, though GPs are not automatically required to accept that person on their list (and health authorities make special arrangements for people who have difficulty finding a doctor who will register them). GPs provide an annual health check for any patient over the age of 75, though some GPs have not provided these checks on a regular basis (National Service Framework for Older People, 2001). A growing number of GPs are employed directly by health authorities (as distinct from holding a contract with them). Each GP practice is also required by the NHS Plan 2000 to publish figures on the numbers of patients removed from their lists.

From the end of the year 2000 all GPs were required to identify anyone amongst their patients who was also a voluntary carer (so be prepared to be asked about your unpaid, or family, caring commitments next time you see your own GP).

Nursing services

Although we may think we know what nurses do, nursing as a profession has sometimes struggled to define a role for itself that stands apart from the work of other colleagues in medicine and social care. Here is one quite widely accepted definition of the nursing task:

'The unique function of the nurse is to assist the individual, sick or well, in the performance of those activities contributing to health or its recovery (or to a peaceful death) that (s)he would perform unaided if (s)he had the necessary strength, will, or knowledge. And to do this in such a way as to help her gain independence as soon as possible' (Henderson, 1966).

However, the NHS Plan 2000 proposes substantial new skills and roles for nurses (with the aim of removing barriers between professional staff in the NHS). For example, (some) nurses will have the right to prescribe a limited range of medicines from 2001. The range of medicines a nurse can prescribe, and the numbers of nurses who can prescribe will be extended, so that by 2004 'a majority of nurses should be able to prescribe' (NHS Plan 2000).

ACTIVITY 22

Getting well, or staying well

- **Thinking about the definition above, is there a difference between helping someone get better and helping them stay well? Write a line or two below; it will help you understand a little more about some of the nursing roles outlined in the remainder of this section. Then read the quotation below ('Trust partnership gives club a real leg-up'); it's a good example of how nursing roles have come to include both getting people better and helping them stay that way.**

'Trust partnership gives club a real leg-up'

'Concern about the number of patients with leg ulcers led to the launch of the Felixstowe Leg Club. Jointly run by nurses from the Felixstowe General Hospital minor injuries unit and community nurses, staff were delighted by its early success. The Club's aim is to help patients with leg problems, particularly ulcers, and to prevent them recurring. Dressings are changed, and lifestyle advice is given to minimise the risk of ulcers recurring. The club is also a social occasion for its members' (Annual Report, Local Health Partnerships NHS Trust, Ipswich, 1999).

Practice nurses and district nurses

Practice nurses are employed by GP practices; district nurses are based at health centres or GP surgeries, but are mostly employed by the local community NHS trust, or by newly established primary care trusts. Though sharing broadly similar skills and responsibilities (eg, wound care and giving injections), practice nurses do most of their work in the surgery or health centre, whilst district nurses visit patients in their own homes, especially important in rural areas where more assessments might need to be done at home. Practice nurses are particularly concerned with maintaining the good health of patients using their surgeries (eg, you may see the practice nurse if you attend a 'Well Woman' or 'Well Man' clinic).

District nurses often carry out the annual health check that all GP practices are required to make on patients who have reached the age of 75. Like GPs, district nurses often hold the key to other services, referring their patient to, say, the community physiotherapist, to Marie Curie nurses, to the dietician or the continence adviser, or advising on the supply of specialist nursing equipment, such as pressure-relieving mattresses. A district nurse will also be involved in helping monitor and prepare an older person's care plan, especially if that person needs very intensive care (such as a night sitting service) or palliative care (ie, they have some form of terminal illness). Some areas also provide a 'twilight' district nursing service between, say, 6pm and 10pm.

Marie Curie nurses

Can provide extra care at home for older people who are seriously ill with cancers. The name Marie Curie honours the twice Nobel Prize-winning scientist who discovered radium. Marie Curie nurses offer a day or night service, working with and relieving carers. This service is arranged through your district nurse (and Marie Curie nurses work within the care plan drawn up by the district nurse). Half the costs of employing a Marie Curie nurse are met by the national charity Marie Curie Cancer Care (the balance is met by the NHS). Marie Curie nurses work with their patients for the last few months or weeks of life.

Macmillan nurses

Macmillan specialist nurses have considerable knowledge, skills and experience in cancer care. They work very closely with other health care professionals, and with social services, supporting patients and their carers, administering some forms of very specialised medication and enabling older patients to stay at home (if that's what they want). They are also expert at controlling pain. Macmillan nurses are based at hospitals and in the community. They are funded and trained for their first three years in post by the national charity Macmillan Cancer Relief. The NHS takes responsibility for their salaries and training from then on. Macmillan nurses work with patients from the point of diagnosis.

Stoma therapists

Stoma therapy is a specialist nursing service for anyone who has had an ileostomy (an operation on a part of the intestine called the ileum), or a colostomy (an operation on the colon, or large intestine). These operations bring part of the ileum or the colon to the surface of the patient's abdomen, making an artificial opening, or 'stoma' that allows for the discharge of body wastes. Stoma therapists are nurses specially trained in the care of these artificial openings. Referral to a stoma therapist will usually be made as part of the discharge planning arrangements as the patient leaves hospital.

Rapid response teams

Rapid response teams (where available) aim to reduce unnecessary admissions of older people to hospital, especially during the winter months, when beds need to be kept free for emergency admissions. The team is likely to include occupational therapists, physiotherapists, district nurses, home carers and hospital staff. The extension of rapid response teams is an important element in the National Service Framework for Older People (2001).

Hospital at home schemes

Some areas offer intensive home care and nursing support for patients recently discharged from hospital after major surgery, or for people who are terminally ill. This sort of support is usually time-limited (eg, up to two weeks after hospital discharge), and can be of particular help to people who live alone, or don't have access to carer support. Some areas also have a 'welcome home' service for people living alone: volunteers go to the patient's home a little before they come back from hospital and light fires, turn on heating systems, stock the larder, clean and dust etc.

Night sitting services

Available in some areas. These services generally involve district nurses and home carers. Some of them are particularly targeted at people with terminal illnesses or at people with high care needs who live with their carer(s).

Community Psychiatric Nurses

Community Psychiatric Nurses (CPNs) may be able to help with some of the problems experienced by people who care for older people with some form of dementia. They may work in conjunction with day hospital or in-patient services provided by your local NHS community trust. CPNs can also work with older people experiencing other kinds of mental health problems, such as depression, and are very likely to be in contact with older people with learning disabilities. Contact CPNs via your GP or social worker.

Continence advisers

Many GP practices have a practice nurse specifically trained to give continence advice and to help supply appropriate aids. Incontinence can be a particularly embarrassing condition, for carers and cared for alike, but there are ways in which the condition can be eased or managed. If there isn't a continence-trained nurse attached to your GP practice, or if you are dealing with a particularly complex continence problem, your doctor can refer you for more specialist help. The community physiotherapist (see below) may also be able to help with appropriate exercises.

Dieticians

Can be of particular help to people with diabetes, people who have been malnourished, people needing some form of food supplements, and people with vitamin deficiency diseases. They can also help people with strokes who have difficulty swallowing. Contact your local dietician through your district nurse or GP.

Speech therapists

May be able to help an older person whose speech and swallowing have been affected by a stroke or other conditions. Contact them via your district nurse or GP.

Community physiotherapists

Can often help maintain an older person's mobility, dignity or independence (see page 55). You'll need a GP's referral to use this service.

Occupational therapists

In some areas, OTs are all employed by the NHS and not by social services. Their work is broadly the same as the work described on page 46.

Wheelchair services

This service is usually run by specially trained OTs, physios and rehabilitation engineers. They can assess and advise on suitable wheelchairs and special seating for older people with disabilities. They can also train older people and their carers in how to use such aids. Referral to this service is through your GP, or an OT or physiotherapist. It is sometimes possible to borrow wheelchairs (or other equipment like commodes, toilet raisers, bed raisers, or walking frames) on short-term loan from your local branch of the British Red Cross Society (see the phone book for their address). In some areas, wheelchairs can only be loaned from the British Red Cross Society on a GP's recommendation.

Aids and equipment

Aids and equipment, such as walking frames, raised toilet seats, and bathing aids, are often supplied from a central store managed jointly by health and social services. It's sometimes possible to visit these stores, and to see equipment on display (which gives the person using that equipment an opportunity, with appropriately skilled advice, to choose an aid(s) for themselves). The prompt provision of aids and equipment, ideally from integrated central stores, is one of the action points set out in the National Service Framework for Older People (2001).

Chiropody services

Older people can be referred to the chiropody and foot-care services provided by NHS community trusts; that is, they don't necessarily have to pay for private chiropody services. In some circumstances, an NHS chiropodist might be able to visit someone at home; talk to a GP or district nurse about using this service. Good chiropody and foot-care services help to prevent falls.

Community dental services

In urban areas, this is sometimes called the borough dental service. It's available for people who are frail or housebound, and although community dentists may be based at a local clinic, they can visit patients at home. It might also be possible for an older person's own dentist to visit them at home. Talk to the patient's dentist or GP about using this service. There's also a specialist dental service provided for people with learning disabilities.

NHS Direct

A nationwide, nurse-led telephone health advisory service designed to relieve some of the pressure on GP or other NHS services. It will also, in time, give information specifically for carers (as part of the Carers' National Strategy). You can ring NHS Direct, 24 hours a day, on 0845 4647 (calls are charged at BT local rates), or consult their website (http://www.doh.gov.uk). The NHS Direct telephone helpline provides confidential healthcare advice and information on:

- What to do if you're feeling ill;
- Health concerns for you and your family;
- Local health services;
- Self-help and support organisations.

(*About NHS Direct*, 2001)

Joint commissioning

This book describes the separate ways in which both health and social services are 'commissioned' or purchased (since both services have different structures and ways of working). 'Commissioning' takes a slightly longer-term view of need than purchasing, which tends to be repeated from year to year. Many health and social services are now jointly planned and jointly funded. This welcome development will be hastened by the work done locally on preparing health improvement programmes or HImPs (see page 51), by the work of primary care groups and trusts, and by the Health Act 1999, which enables health and social service departments to pool their budgets, to employ staff who have previously worked in one or other department, and to provide services together through a single organisation (what the NHS Plan 2000 describes as 'care trusts').

ACTIVITY 23

Community health services

- **Write a sentence or two below (or at the back of this book) picking out any services an older person in your care might benefit from but does not get at present. Show those notes to your line manager or supervisor.**

Welfare benefits

The probability is that almost anyone you care for will receive some form of welfare benefit, for example, the state retirement pension; you may also be entitled to claim welfare benefits for yourself. *This section will help S/NVQ candidates find the underpinning knowledge needed for Care Level 2 Unit Y1, 'Enable individuals to manage their domestic and personal resources'.*

What are welfare benefits?

Any form of cash benefit the state gives to retired people, people on low incomes, the sick and unemployed, families with children, people with disabilities, and people who care at home for someone with disabilities. There are three broad categories of welfare benefits:

- Those intended to replace earnings – these are benefits that compensate anyone unable to work because of sickness, disability, unemployment, pregnancy, retirement, or caring responsibilities. Many of these benefits are not subject to any form of means test (ie, they can always be paid, no matter what level of income or capital a claimant has); but some, such as retirement and widows' pensions, depend on the claimant's National Insurance record (or her husband's).
- Those which compensate for extra costs, such as living with a disability.
- Those which help alleviate poverty, eg Income Support (also called the Minimum Income Guarantee for pensioners), council tax benefit and housing benefit.

How can I find out about these benefits?

You can sometimes pick up a relevant leaflet in your local post office, though there's no guarantee you'll find the one you want. In England, Wales and Scotland, you can also contact the Benefits Agency direct (their local office address will be in the phone book), though not for queries about National Insurance contributions (which now go to the Inland Revenue) or unemployment benefits (ask your local Jobcentre about these). You should also bear in mind that in some parts of London the Benefits Agency office is basically a 'caller point', with the work being done in other parts of the country. If you're enquiring about benefits for people who are sick, disabled or carers, then you can also call the Benefit Enquiry Line (BEL). Their freephone number is 0800 882200, and they are open from 8.30am to 6.30pm Monday to Friday, and from 9am to 1pm on Saturdays.

Arrangements in Northern Ireland are a little different. Welfare benefits there, though paid at the same rate, and under the same circumstances, as benefits elsewhere in the United Kingdom, are administered by the Social Security Agency. Their freephone Benefit Enquiry Line is on 0800 220674, is also available for queries on sickness and disability benefits etc, and is open from 9am to 5pm, Mondays to Fridays.

Alternatively you can contact the welfare rights adviser at your local social services or social work department, a carers' group you belong to or the local Citizens Advice Bureau. You could also call the Age Concern Information Line, on 0800 00 99 66, from 7am to 7pm, seven days a week, to ask for a range of free factsheets, including one on money benefits for older people.

Two important benefits that are not administered by the Benefits Agency are housing benefit and council tax benefit ('rate rebate' in Northern Ireland). These are benefits administered by local councils. You can find their name and address by looking on your own council tax demands (assuming, of course, that you and the person you care for live in the same council district). You'll also find that some welfare benefits (eg, Attendance Allowance, Disability Living Allowance, Invalid Care Allowance) are not administered by local Benefits Agency offices but through one, or a number, of specialised offices that deal with the country as a whole. Your local Benefits Agency will give you an appropriate application form and a pre-paid envelope.

Should I encourage someone to claim welfare benefits?

Undoubtedly yes; a great tragedy of the welfare state is that so many benefits are not taken up by those entitled to them. Almost every benefit has to be claimed; that is, it isn't paid automatically. Reforms to the welfare system that trigger benefits are still some way off. Though many retirement pensioners are amongst the poorest people in the country, there are still not enough older people taking up benefits they could be claiming. Do encourage them to take up what is, after all, their entitlement, not a charitable 'hand-out'. What follows is a brief description of some benefits that seem particularly applicable to older people and their carers. A fuller description of them all can be found in the *Disability Rights Handbook*, price £12.50 post-free (2001/2), the Age Concern guide *Your Rights: A guide to money benefits for older people*, price £4.50 in 2001, or the Child Poverty Action Group's *Welfare Benefits Handbook*, price £22.00 for two volumes (2001/2). You can buy all three benefit guides from the organisations concerned (their addresses and phone numbers can be found in Appendix 1, 'Useful addresses', pages 104–117). Age Concern England also has a number of free fact-sheets on welfare benefits (see page 117 for further details).

ACTIVITY 24

Unclaimed benefits

- **Can you think of anyone in your care who might be entitled to benefits they haven't claimed? How might you encourage them to make a claim? List some suggestions below.**

State retirement pensions

The state retirement pension can be claimed from age 60, for women, and age 65, for men (though from 2010 the age at which women claim their state retirement pension will be gradually increased, so that by 2020 both men and women will claim their pensions at 65). There are basically three types of state retirement pension:

Category A pensions are normally based on the claimant's National Insurance contributions record. To claim a full Category A pension, you need to have paid National Insurance contributions for roughly nine out of every ten years since your sixteenth birthday (or to have been 'credited' with contributions because you were sick, unemployed or in full-time education). Allowances for dependants, such as children, or someone looking after the children, can be added to the Category A pension.

Category B pensions are generally paid to women over pension age who are, or have been, married. Category B pensions are based on the contribution record of your spouse, or former spouse. If he didn't pay his contributions in full, the pension is reduced accordingly. Category B pensions are paid at about two-thirds the rate of Category A pensions.

Category D pensions are non-contributory, and paid at the same rate as Category B pensions, but only to people over the age of 80. They were originally designed for people who were too old to have paid sufficient contributions into the state retirement scheme.

There is generally no limit to the amount that someone can earn whilst claiming the state retirement pension (though the pension counts as income for tax purposes). If you work beyond retirement age, you can put off the age at which you claim your pension for up to five years (till age 70 for men, and 65 for women, but no later than that).

For anyone who has not paid into a contracted out private pension scheme, the basic rate of pension can be 'topped up' by SERPS (the State Earnings Related Pension Scheme). There is also a graduated retirement benefit (a scheme that ran from 1961 to 1974), though the weekly benefits from this scheme are relatively small.

Provided you apply four months before the date you are due to retire, the Inland Revenue will give you a pension forecast. Ask for leaflet BR19 at your local Benefits Agency office (or its equivalent from the Social Security Agency in Northern Ireland).

Income Support

Is intended to provide for basic living expenses for the claimant and their family. It can be paid on its own for someone with no other income, or used to top up some other kind of benefit, such as the state retirement pension. If someone doesn't have much money coming in, it's always worth checking to see if they qualify for income support.

There are several key tests that anyone claiming Income Support has to 'pass', for example:

- they must be in Great Britain, and 'habitually resident' in the UK, the Channel Islands, the Isle of Man or the Republic of Ireland;
- they must not be working for more than 16 hours per week;
- they must not have capital of more than £12,000 (for someone over the age of 60), or £18,500 for someone living permanently in a residential home (April 2001);
- they must be in one of the categories of people eligible for income support (eg, a carer, anyone incapable of work, and anyone aged over 60).

Anyone who passes these tests is entitled to Income Support, provided their income, worked out under IS rules, is 'less than the amount the law says you need to live on'. The exact amount that anyone needs to live on (reviewed by Parliament each year) is worked out in three parts. These are called:

- personal allowances – for a single claimant, a couple, or dependent children;
- premiums – a flat-rate addition if the claimant satisfies certain conditions;
- housing costs – generally the cost of mortgage interest repayments.

It's the *premiums* that are so important to older or disabled people, or their carers, since they boost the amount that anyone 'needs to live on'. There is a premium for people aged 60 or over, and a disability premium for disabled people under 60 who fulfil certain conditions. There is also a severe disability premium (which certain people receiving Attendance Allowance or Disability Living Allowance will qualify for), and a carer's premium (paid if someone or their partner receives the Invalid Care Allowance, or has an entitlement to ICA).

Another important feature of Income Support is that it triggers certain other benefits, such as free prescriptions for people under 60, dental treatment, help with hospital fares, and additional help with the cost of buying spectacles.

To claim Income Support, ask the Benefits Office for form SP1 (for pensioners) or form A1 (for everyone else). It's rather a lengthy form, but can be completed by someone else on the claimant's behalf.

Attendance Allowance

A tax-free benefit payable to someone aged 65 and over who is severely disabled, mentally or physically, and needs either supervision or help with their personal care (such as washing, dressing or using the toilet). What matters with Attendance Allowance is the help that someone needs, whether or not they get that help, and whether or not they live alone.

There are two rates of Attendance Allowance, with the higher rate payable to people who need help and/or supervision during the night *and* during the day, and the lower rate payable to people who need help and/or supervision during the day, *or* during the night.

Attendance Allowance is payable only to people over 65, 'ordinarily resident' in the UK, who have needed care and supervision for at least six months, or who are terminally ill (in which case the six-month condition does not apply).

People claiming Attendance Allowance are not normally asked to have an independent medical examination, since the Benefits Agency 'adjudicator' will normally have sufficient information from the application form (which is often filled in by the claimant's GP, nurse or social worker).

To make a claim for Attendance Allowance, ring the Benefit Enquiry Line on 0800 882200 (0800 220674 in Northern Ireland) and ask for the Attendance Allowance Claim Pack (DS2).

Disability Living Allowance

The Disability Living Allowance (DLA) is a benefit for both children and adults who need help looking after themselves, or help in getting around (what used to be called a mobility allowance). It's not taxable, and doesn't depend on anyone's National Insurance contribution records. You can also claim DLA while continuing in full-time employment.

There are two 'components' to DLA, a care component and a mobility component. The care component is divided into three rates of payment. The top two payment rates are the same as the two rates of payment used for Attendance Allowance. To pass the care component tests requires roughly the same needs for help and supervision as Attendance Allowance claims require. The higher-rate mobility component is paid to people who cannot walk, or are virtually unable to walk, are blind and deaf, or to certain people who have a 'severe mental impairment'. The lower rate is paid to anyone who cannot use an unfamiliar route outdoors without 'guidance and supervision' from someone else.

Anyone claiming DLA must be ordinarily resident in the UK; must have been disabled for three months before they start to receive the allowance (and likely to be disabled for six months after the claim); must pass the 'disability tests' outlined above; and must be aged under 65 when they first make their claim (though, once claimed, DLA is payable beyond someone's 65th birthday).

Special conditions apply to people on renal dialysis and people who are terminally ill. Like Attendance Allowance, certain rates of DLA can trigger someone's entitlement to other benefits, such as the severe disability premium for Income Support.

To make a claim for DLA, ask the Benefits Agency for the DLA Claim Pack (DLA1), or telephone one of the Benefit Enquiry Lines (0800 882200 or, for Northern Ireland, 0800 220674). Backdated claims begin from the date of that initial enquiry to the Benefits Agency or the BEL. Remember that if someone other than the Benefits Agency, such as the Citizens Advice Bureau, gives out a DLA Claim Pack, that claim can be backdated only to the date when the completed form DLA1 is received by the Benefits Agency (rather than the date when the form was first given out).

Invalid Care Allowance

Invalid Care Allowance (ICA) is a benefit for people under 65 who regularly spend more than 35 hours each week caring for someone who is severely disabled. To claim ICA, you must be:

- aged 16–64;
- ordinarily resident in the UK;
- not in full-time education;

and you must be spending more than 35 hours per week looking after someone who receives either:

- the DLA care component (at the middle or higher rates);
- Attendance Allowance (at either the higher or the lower rate);
- certain forms of war disablement or industrial injuries pension.

You cannot claim ICA if your take-home pay is more than £72.00 per week (2001), though some allowance is made for the costs of paying someone else to look after the person being cared for whilst you are at work. You will not receive payment if some of the other benefits you get come to more than your ICA (though you can claim ICA as well as Attendance Allowance or DLA). Claiming ICA also means that you receive the carer's premium in means-tested benefits.

You claim ICA by filling in form DS700, which you can get from the local Benefits Agency office.

Housing and council tax benefits

These benefits are to help people with low incomes or on Income Support to pay their rent and council tax (or their rates in Northern Ireland). For the most part, you cannot claim either benefit if you have capital of more than £16,000.

'HB' and 'CTB' are mostly administered by local authorities, or the Northern Ireland Housing Executive/Rate Collection Agency (which then reclaim the money involved from central government). Anyone on Income Support will gain from HB and CTB; do remind them of this entitlement.

Preserved rights

Anyone who entered a residential care home (but not a local authority care home) prior to April 1993 'preserved' their rights to any Income Support payments they received to help with the payment of care home fees. The problem with this arrangement has been that Income Support payments have not necessarily kept pace with the increase in care home fees (leading to considerable anxiety for the residents involved). From April 2002, local authorities will take responsibility for the assessment, care, management and financial support of people who previously had Preserved Rights, ie, care home payments made on their behalf become the responsibility of a local authority, not the Benefits Agency. In the meantime, it should be possible for local authorities to support older people with preserved rights who are threatened with eviction to stay in their existing residential care homes (The NHS Plan (2000), The Government's response to the Royal Commission on Long Term Care).

3 Looking after yourself

This part of the guide begins with a very brief description of some rights you have as an employee. If you need further advice on employment matters, if you think you may have grounds to claim compensation for injuries suffered at work, or should you find yourself in any kind of dispute with your employer, then it is a wise precaution to seek advice from people who understand such things in detail, for example the personnel section where you work, your trade union representative, or a solicitor specialising in employment law.

Contracts of employment and induction

Every employee has a contract of employment; it's something you sign when you first accept your employer's offer of a job. Do keep this document safely. It contains some very important information, like the hours you must work, your rates of pay, what holidays you are entitled to, your commitments, if any, to a pension scheme, your rights to join a trade union, and which, if any, of those unions your employer 'recognises' when it comes to negotiations over pay etc. You won't have a contract of employment if your employer claims that you are self-employed. Don't forget that in these circumstances you are responsible for making your own income tax payments and National Insurance contributions (as well as any contributions to a pension fund).

It's also good practice for every new employee to be given some form of 'induction' programme (so that the new job is properly explained to you, you know what your rights and responsibilities are, and where to find what you need). If any part of your induction programme has been neglected or rushed, then go back to your line manager and ask if they can make time to explain things to you; you cannot be blamed for not doing something properly if you were never told how to do things correctly in the first place.

Disciplinary and grievance procedures

Every employer should have some form of disciplinary and grievance procedure. A copy of each procedure is sometimes sent in the same envelope as your contract of employment (so keep them somewhere that's easy to get to if you need them). Alternatively, you might have discussed such things when you first met your line manager, or as part of your induction programme.

Disciplinary proceedings may be used if your employer thinks you have done something against their procedures. Great care should be taken in these circumstances to hear your side of the story fairly, and to keep the details of what anyone may have said about you in the strictest confidence. Disciplinary proceedings might also be used if the standard of your work seems to be slipping, and there's no easy explanation for why this might be happening.

Disciplinary proceedings are never comfortable, but nor do people being disciplined always get dismissed; handled well, a disciplinary 'hearing' should be concerned not just with the rights and wrongs of the matter in hand, but with finding the right kinds of help to get someone back to the proper level of performance. Trade unions will usually represent a member involved in any kind of dispute with their employer.

Grievance procedures are also there for your protection. Trade unions can help their members in this situation too. Grievance procedures can be used if you think your employer has acted unfairly towards you, and the matter cannot be resolved in discussions with whomever you think has not acted properly. 'Taking out a grievance' means your employer has to investigate the matter thoroughly; whoever carries out that investigation has to be independent of the person you are complaining about. There should always be an appeals procedure available to you if you are dissatisfied with the first investigation of your grievance.

Health and safety procedures

Health and safety procedures play a very important part in looking after yourself at work. Employers should give you a copy of their health and safety procedures along with your contract of employment, or as part of your induction training. You should expect to be trained or advised, for example, on what to do if fire breaks out; how to lift without injuring yourself or others; how to deal with bodily fluids; and what you can safely do when working in a service user's home (eg, the care you need to take when using any kind of electrical appliance). If you are unfortunate enough to hurt yourself at work, you may have to complete an accident report form. Many large organisations keep a careful record of where and when accidents occur; serious accidents have to be recorded on a special form provided by the Health and Safety Executive (HSE). Employers who don't keep accurate records of all accidents or injuries that happen to staff or residents, or who don't train their staff in health and safety procedures, may be held responsible for failing to provide a safe working or living environment. HSE Inspectors have a right to see the accident report book, and any other safety records (Health and Safety at Work Act 1984, Section 20[k]). Always remember that you are personally responsible for taking reasonable care of your own health and safety at work, and the health and safety of anyone else who could be affected by anything you do, or forget to do (Health and Safety at Work Act 1984, Section 7).

Equal opportunities

Any form of abuse or discrimination on grounds of race, ethnicity or religion is simply not acceptable in a multi-cultural society, and may also be illegal (Race Relations Act 1976 and the Race Relations [Northern Ireland] Order 1997). Racial abuse is something you must respond to as it happens (or the moment to say something is probably lost). Such remarks must never be ignored and must always be challenged – whatever your own racial background. It may be tempting to think that older people who make racially abusive remarks 'don't really mean it', or that 'things were different in their day', or that 'you can't really expect people of 80-plus to change their ways'. Whilst anyone may be entitled to their opinions, there is no need, and really no excuse, for being offensive. If such remarks go unchallenged, they begin to look acceptable, with the serious possibility that others may suffer too. There is also a risk that if racist behaviour is ignored, we start to think of older people as childlike and unable to control their own behaviour. Many employers have clear codes of conduct about racist and discriminatory behaviour on the part of staff and service users (something you should also be told about as part of your induction). Any employer who discriminates against someone solely on the basis of that person's disability (for instance, refusing them a job, or promotion) commits an offence under the Disability Discrimination Act 1995.

Many employers also have clear codes of conduct about sexual harassment. Whilst a colleague who harasses you may be disciplined, sexual harassment of a female carer by, say, a male service user is less likely to be covered by your employer's codes of conduct. If ever you find yourself in this unpleasant situation, report what's happening to your line manager at the earliest opportunity. Don't think that you just have to handle it, or that (s)he doesn't really mean it. There's a real risk that things will get even worse, for both of you, when such behaviour goes unreported. Covering up for men (or women) who behave in this way denies them help when they may need it most.

Gifts from service users

Many of the organisations you are likely to work for will have strict rules about taking gifts from service users; for example, the maximum value of any gift you are allowed to accept from a service user may be as little as £5.00. Induction programmes or 'packages' should explain your employer's policies about receiving gifts (if not, then ask your line manager at the earliest opportunity about accepting gifts from service users). In practice, refusing a gift can be very difficult, especially if it is a genuine expression of someone's affection for you, or the regard in which they hold you. But think of things this way. Giving gifts can sometimes be a way of trying to influence people. Some people forget they have given something away that had been of importance to them. Whether or not anyone has the 'right' to give something away can also be a very touchy subject (especially if there are members of the older person's family who want to influence the way their relative handles money or property). It's always a good idea to explain the rules you have to work to whenever you suspect a service user plans to give you something, say, at Christmas time, or around other major festivals like Divali.

Complaints procedures

Complaints procedures can change things in any organisation only if they are used. Complaints should not be resisted; they can be a very important way of improving services. As a general rule, however, it is better to resolve complaints informally; putting things right first time can save a lot of work, worry, and anxiety later on. Always inform your line manager if you think a complaint may be made against you, for whatever reason. If you belong to a trade union, their representative might also be able to help you. You should have nothing to fear if the service you gave met the standard required.

Every health authority, NHS Trust, primary care group, primary care trust, and social services department (and many voluntary organisations too) will have a formal complaints procedure. All these organisations should make it easy for service users and others to find out how they can make a complaint (it should be the kind of information that's available across the counter at your local hospital, surgery, or social services department, for instance). The importance of making complaints (as you read at the start of the previous paragraph) is that it helps the organisation concerned to find out what people think about the quality of its services; ie, it's another way of giving service users a 'voice' in the sorts of services available to them. The NHS Plan 2000 has some interesting proposals for giving people who use health and (some) social care services 'more say in their own treatment and more influence over the way [a service] works' (NHS Plan 2000). For example:

- Letters about an individual patient's care will be copied to the patient as of right.
- A new NHS Charter (due 2001) will replace the current Patient's Charter. 'It will make clear how people can access NHS services,

what the NHS commitment is to patients, and the rights and responsibilities patients have within the NHS' (NHS Plan 2000).

- All NHS trusts, primary care groups and primary care trusts will have to ask patients for their views on the services they've received, and the results of the National Patients Survey will be used to decide 'how much cash [the Trusts etc] get' (NHS Plan 2000).
- Residential care homes will be expected to seek the views of residents on improvements the home could make, and to show, each year, how many of those improvements have been put in place.
- Older people will be represented on Commission for Health Improvement inspection teams (as 'lay' people currently are on local authority inspection teams) to ensure that 'older people's dignity and interests are fully taken into account' (NHS Plan 2000).
- By 2002, a Patient Advocacy and Liaison Service (PALS) will be established in every NHS Trust, starting with the major hospitals. Based on a successful scheme in Brighton, PALS will be found near hospital reception areas, for example, and will act as a 'welcoming point' for patients and carers. As patient advocates, they will also have direct access to the Chief Executive of any Trust, and the power to negotiate an immediate solution to any problem where appropriate.

Disclosure (or 'whistle blowing')

One of the reasons why abuses in care practice have sometimes been slow to come to light is that powerful people try to cover them up, or colleagues are very loath to tell what they know. If your organisation has a 'disclosure' policy (and many do), then try to read it through. Deciding to 'split' on a colleague or a manager may be one of the hardest decisions you ever have to make. Here are three points to remember if ever you have to 'tell':

- Colleagues may want you to believe that you got them into trouble. The truth may be that they got themselves into trouble by doing something they knew to be wrong.
- The people you look after need help because they cannot arrange their own lives in ways they would want. Professional care workers have a 'duty of care' to anyone they look after – it means such people have to be properly cared for. Abuse of any sort betrays that trust.

- 'Whistle blowers' are starting to get the protection they deserve. There is a Public Interest Disclosure Act (1998) to protect workers who 'speak out in good faith and the public interest'. There has also been an increase (up to £50,000) in the compensation payable to brave people who risk their careers by speaking out and are then unfairly dismissed from their jobs. The organisation Public Concern at Work (see Appendix 1, 'Useful addresses', page 108) will also help anyone who feels they need to whistle blow on some improper practice at work.

ACTIVITY 25

'Whistle blowing'

- **How might you feel if you had to 'blow the whistle' (ie, 'tell') on someone at work? Write a sentence or two starting, 'What I would do if I found someone doing something wrong and couldn't persuade them to stop is ...'**

Carer-sensitive employment policies

There are some very good reasons why any employer should make their employment practices more sensitive to the needs of carers (not forgetting that care workers often care for others voluntarily).

- At least 24 per cent of all adults aged between 45 and 64 care voluntarily. Any group of employees, especially in the caring services, will include an appreciable number of people in this age group.
- If carers leave employment because they cannot see any alternative to giving up their jobs, the company will lose their experience, and

will have to train whomever takes their place. It can cost a great deal (perhaps as much as a year's salary) to get new staff members working to the same standard as more experienced colleagues.
- Equality of opportunity, or being fair to everyone, is something most employees value. Word gets around. Companies with good employment policies are more likely to attract good staff.

As you may know from your own experience, there are at least three good reasons why caring for elderly or disabled people is different from caring for children and young people:

- The need for care, eg, when someone suffers a stroke, occurs suddenly. There may be greater warning when children or young people are taken seriously ill.
- Caring for someone with dementia can be a very unpredictable experience; you never quite know what to expect. Looking after children may lead to fewer of these unexpected incidents.
- As children grow older, they become more self-sufficient, and need less care over time. An older person's condition may deteriorate, so that they need more care over time.

This suggests that employers who are sensitive to the needs of carers on their staff should:

- not put pressure on them to do additional hours, make it difficult for them to leave work on time, or fail to give advance notice if someone is required to work overtime, or attend a course or meeting away from home;
- develop the sorts of flexible leave arrangements that either make it possible for carers to deal with crises (eg, an allocation of unpaid leave carers can take each year), or make it easier for them to return to work after a caring break (eg, a guarantee they can return to the same or a similar job within a certain period);
- make it possible for carers to discuss their caring responsibilities comfortably, and in confidence (men, in particular, can find it very hard to admit to having caring responsibilities, thinking that any admission they might not cope with extra work responsibilities would harm their future promotion prospects);

- support the Government's commitment to 'Work Life Balance': ie, employees shouldn't be forced to work excessive hours at the expense of their family commitments.

If you have caring responsibilities your employer is not aware of, do think hard about discussing them with someone who could help, such as a line manager. You might then find it easier to take time out if and when next you need it (though don't forget that all employees have a legal right to take a reasonable period of time of work to deal with an emergency involving a dependant, ACAS 2000).

S/NVQ candidates for Care Level 2 awards should note they will be asked to include a copy of their employer's equal opportunities, and health and safety policies in their 'portfolio'.

Further learning

If you've enjoyed reading this guide, you might have been encouraged to look into opportunities for further learning. You do challenging and responsible jobs. This is what the English White Paper on *Modernising Social Services* (1998) says about work in the caring services: 'people who work in social care are called on to respond to some of the most demanding, often distressing and intractable human problems' (paragraph 5.2, p 84).

Work on any caring activity takes both courage and compassion, often in equal measure. None of us can afford to sit back and think we've 'cracked' whatever caring job we do. We need to learn from each set of new experiences; that's what 'life-long learning' (or 'CPD' – Continuous Professional Development) is all about.

If you're thinking, rightly, that training opportunities for staff in residential and day care services have been left behind, then take heart. The fact that from October 2001, we have a new General Social Care Council (like the registration bodies that nurses already have) means that training for day and residential staff cannot continue to be the rather hit-and-miss affair it has been up to now. No one can be required to hold any qualification (and in time all care staff will need a suitable qualification for their post) unless the training is there to help them get that qualification. If all that sounds frightening, then rest assured, the sorts of qualifications carers will need are not going to be old-fashioned pen-and-paper examinations, but assessments of the skills and knowledge they can show 'on the job'. As many of us know, it's never too late to learn; the more experienced you become, the better able you should be to demonstrate your skills and knowledge in practice. This section outlines some of the training opportunities available to you now.

A good starting point for working out your own learning needs is to begin with what you have learned from reading this guide. Here are four 'steps' that will help you fit that learning into your own work setting. As you can see, the third of those steps includes discussion with your line manager. If you are employed, then you may have regular meetings with your line manager for 'supervision', or 'consultation'. Always try to approach those meetings constructively. They are often the best way of clarifying any problems you have in practice (which also makes them an excellent way to learn).

Activity 26

Applying what you've learned

1. **Write down what you knew about community care for older people and their carers before you started reading the guide.**
2. **Work out what you thought you would gain from reading the guide, and share this with your line manager, or someone from a carers' organisation both of you belong to.**
3. **In discussions with your manager, or your colleague, work out what it is you need to do differently now that you've read the guide.**
4. **Wait till you've put those changes into practice, and then ask your manager or your colleague for their honest opinion on how well you're doing.**

You'll now find a brief note of training and learning opportunities that could be relevant to the job you do. The chapter finishes with a brief revision exercise.

Scottish and National Vocational Qualifications

The care sector was one of the first to move into Scottish Vocational Qualifications (SVQs) and National Vocational Qualifications (NVQs); the first awards were made in 1990. Some of you may already be S/NVQ 'candidates', which is why parts of this guide refer to the 'knowledge evidence' you need for particular Care Level 2 Units.

Every S/NVQ is based on National Occupational Standards. The standards are a measure of how well caring tasks should be done. Each S/NVQ candidate is assessed against these standards (which are called 'competences'). Your assessor will always be someone experienced in your kind of work (and may be one of your line managers). Assessors observe candidates 'on the job'. They ask questions about the way a job is being done; and they look at other evidence that shows how well candidates understand their job, starting with what they have put in their 'portfolio'. Portfolios are where you can store 'paper' evidence, such as press cuttings, documents your employer needs you to understand (eg, health and safety at work procedures), and evidence that comes from what you've read (eg, the Activities in this guide). Tape recordings and video recordings can go into portfolios too. By and large, assessors will act only once the candidate is ready to have their work assessed.

There are three 'levels' of S/NVQs in Care; the higher the level, the more complicated the work you'll be assessed on. There is currently one 'integrated' care award at Level 2, three awards at Level 3, and one award at Level 4. Each award has a number of units, some of which you must complete, whilst others can be chosen from a list of 'optional' units.

How do I find out about S/NVQs?

You should start by asking your employer; many organisations have some access to an S/NVQ Assessment Centre. Larger organisations may have someone who acts as their S/NVQ adviser. The likelihood is you'll be offered training to help you reach the S/NVQ standards (assuming, that is, that you need it). Don't forget that 50 per cent of all residential care staff in adult services in England are expected to hold an appropriate NVQ at levels 2 and 3 by 2005 (*Modernising the Social Care Workforce*,TOPSS, 2000). The NHS is also committed to providing 'dedicated training' to NVQ level 2 and 3 for support staff like healthcare assistants (as an alternative to opening them an Individual Learning Account of £150 per year).

If you can't get information on S/NVQs at work, then go to your local Learning and Skills Council. You'll find its phone number in the business section of the local telephone directory.

Other learning opportunities

It may be that you've not long left school, in which case you may want to think about a **modern apprenticeship** in care. These are available to anyone aged 18–24 (ie, up to your 25th birthday). Modern apprenticeships include an NVQ at Level 3, along with training in a number of other 'key' skills, for example, numeracy, IT (information technology), and communication skills. There may be similar opportunities for older people who are unemployed. Contact your local Chamber of Commerce, Training and Enterprise for details.

It may also be that you want time to work on other skills before putting yourself forward for S/NVQ assessment; for example, your first priority might be brushing up some IT skills. **Individual Learning Credits** (worth £150 per person) open your 'learning account'. This is part of the government's 'University for Industry' programme (UfI). Your learning account pays for training you buy in consultation with a training adviser, provided you are prepared to put £25 of your own money into the account, and provided you are not claiming Jobseeker's Allowance. You may be able in this way to buy training you can do at home, via digital TV, or 'on line' through your computer; employers might also be prepared to put money into your learning account (which helps you buy more training relevant to your needs). To get started in the UfI, ring freephone Learning Direct on 0800 100

900, or contact your local TEC, or Chamber of Commerce, Training and Enterprise. You can, of course, use your Individual Learning Credits to help pay S/NVQ registration and tuition fees, though the Credit may not cover all the fees involved. As you 'draw' on your account, you'll be given vouchers you can spend with approved training providers; you can also spend up to £50 on careers advice and guidance, or on local authority registered childcare arrangements. One of the recommendations in the NHS Plan 2000 is that individual learning accounts of £150 per year should be opened for all NHS support staff, like healthcare assistants, provided they are not already involved in 'dedicated training' for an NVQ at levels two or three (NHS Plan 2000).

Another opportunity your employer may offer are the City and Guilds Affinity Awards, very similar to S/NVQs but at a slightly lower level. Voluntary carers may like to know that in conjunction with the Carers National Association, City and Guilds are preparing an award(s) directly relevant to them (though as yet there is no firm indication as to when that award(s) might be ready).

Distance learning

If you're already working on S/NVQs but cannot get to formal training events, or if you work for an employer who cannot make such training opportunities available to you (or if you're someone who wants another string to your training 'bow'), there are a number of distance learning packs available you can work on at home, or with groups of colleagues at work. 'Distance learning' means you, or the group, works its own way through activities and exercises, or video and audio tapes, usually with the help of a tutor who may comment on the work you're doing. Amongst the largest suppliers of distance learning materials is the National Extension College (NEC); their address and phone number are listed in Appendix 1. You'll also find that Age Concern England have a number of publications, like this one, that are cross-referenced or directly relevant to Level 2 and 3 Awards in Care.

A distance learning alternative is the Open University (OU), especially if you're thinking of working towards a diploma or a degree.

No formal qualifications are needed to join any OU undergraduate programme. One starting point could be the one-year OU Certificate in Health and Social Care. A number of the OU health and social welfare courses are relevant to S/NVQs, and some carry English National Board (ENB) credits that nurses can use for post-registration training. The OU's Prospectus Request Line is listed in Appendix 1 (page 107).

Keeping up to date

Some forthcoming changes

October 2001: Nursing care will be provided free of charge in nursing homes and residential care homes.

October 2001: The General Social Care Council (GSSC) is formally set up. The GSSC will develop codes of practice for the social care workforce in England, and their employers, and will begin to register the social care workforce (in the way that nurses and other professional staff in the NHS must already be registered).

October 2001: All NHS Departments must have assessed their policies to ensure that no decisions are made on the basis of age alone.

March 2002: At least 40,000 extra people should be receiving intermediate care services, which promote rehabilitation and supported discharge from hospital, compared to the numbers of people receiving such services in 1999/2000.

April 2002: The National Commission for Care Standards (NCCS) takes over inspection and registration responsibilities from local authorities in England. The NCCS will register and inspect residential care homes and domiciliary care services (amongst other services).

April 2002: New national minimum standards apply to practice in all care homes for older people in England. The National Commission for Care Standards will apply these standards.

April 2002: The system of 'Preserved Rights' for older people who entered independent-sector residential care homes before April

1993 comes to an end. Local authorities will now be responsible for the assessment, care, management and financial support of people who previously had preserved rights.

April 2002: All health and social care services must have a single assessment process in place.

2002: By 2002, a Patient Advocacy and Liaison Service (PALS) will be established in every NHS Trust.

April 2003: All local health care providers (health, social services and the independent sector) should have procedures in place to reduce the risk of older people falling.

April 2003: All health and social care organisations should have systems in place to 'explore' the sorts of experiences people have in using those services.

March 2004: At least 150,000 extra people should be receiving intermediate care services, which promote rehabilitation and supported discharge from hospital, compared to the numbers of people receiving such services in 1999/2000.

April 2004: Primary care trusts should have similar systems in place to 'explore' the experience of people using their services.

April 2004: All primary care groups are expected to have become primary care trusts.

2005: 50 per cent of all residential care staff in adult services are expected to hold an appropriate NVQ at levels 2 or 3.

It's very important that care workers try to keep abreast with changes in the health and social care services. The better informed you are, the better able you are to give accurate advice to people you are caring for. If you are able to use the Internet, then the Department of Health's website (http://www.doh.gov.uk) and the King's Fund website (http://www.kingsfund.org.uk) are useful sources of accurate and up-to-date information. The Department of Health website also has a service for people with learning disabilities (at the time of writing, April 2001, that service is relatively small, but it is likely to be expanded in future).

Some revision exercises

One way of working out what it is you've learned from reading this guide is to go back over all or some of the Activities. To make that task easier for you, Activities 2–26 are set out below. Look up the answers you gave earlier as you worked through each Activity. If you've not used them already, the blank pages that follow may help you jot down any notes you want to make. (For Activity 1, see page x, since its purpose is for you to tell us how well this guide met your objectives, not to help with your revision.)

ACTIVITY 2

Spot the sectors

- Think of at least three services an older person you are caring for currently receives. Put each of the services you have chosen in the right 'sector'. Then see if you can think of any differences in the way those services are financed. You can write your answers in the space below or in the blank pages at the back of this book.

ACTIVITY 3

The legal framework

- Why do you think carers should have some knowledge of the law? Use the space below to write down your answers.

ACTIVITY 4

The NHS and Community Care Act 1990

- Can you work out what the connections are between Sir Roy Griffiths' recommendations and the Act itself? The three words 'needs', 'wants' and 'choice' may give you a clue. Write your answers in the space below.

ACTIVITY 5

Asking for help

- See if you can complete the following sentence for yourself. Older people might have difficulty asking for help because they don't know what to ask for; they don't speak English as a first language; they are frightened of ...

ACTIVITY 6

Knocking on the care manager's door

- Very few older people refer themselves to social services departments. They are referred by their GP, by other agencies or by their family and friends. Do care workers have a role in helping people overcome their fear of 'officialdom'? Jot down your answer below.

Activity 7

When to speak out, and when to keep quiet

- Try to imagine yourself being present during an older person's community care assessment. Write a few lines in your own words about what you might want to say, and when you would say it. Use the blank pages at the back of this book if that's easier for you.

Activity 8

Finding out about eligibility crieria

- Where would you go to find out about eligibility criteria or the continuing care criteria used in the National Health Service? Jot down some good starting points below. Here are some clues to get you going: your line manager should know where the criteria for your area can be found, but if you are working on your own, try your authority's Community Care Plan, or the annual reports published each year by the NHS Trusts in your area – there should be copies in your public library.

Activity 9

Using the care plan

- Many of you will be working to at least one care plan, and probably to several (one for each of the people you work with). What is the importance of the care plan for you as a care worker? Look back to 'Why do I need to know about them?' for some extra clues. Try to write two or three sentences on the importance of care plans below, including a line or two on the importance of person-centred planning.

ACTIVITY 10

Keeping good records

- How do you think your own records could be improved? Write a sentence or two below.

ACTIVITY 11

Review meetings

- Think of a review meeting you might have attended/could attend in future. How did you/might you feel before and after that review? Jot down a sentence or two.

ACTIVITY 12

Contracts

- Can you think of any way in which a contract your agency holds affects your day-to-day work with service users? Make some notes below or on the blank pages at the back of this book.

Activity 13

Empowerment

- In your experience, how do older people become 'disempowered'? Write a sentence or two below.

Activity 14

Advocacy in practice

- Think back to a meeting where you had to (or would have liked to) speak up for someone whose voice wouldn't otherwise be heard. Which principles applied to what you said or would have liked to say? Make a brief note showing how the principles fitted what you said. Use the space below, or preferably the blank pages at the back of this book.

Activity 15

Carers' isolation

- Make a note below of anyone in your immediate neighbourhood you think of as a voluntary carer. How many of those people are in regular contact with the caring services?

ACTIVITY 16

The Carer's Charter

- Look out a copy of the Carer's Charter for the area where you live or work. Any carers' association will probably have a copy they can send you, or you can ask if your line manager has a copy. Check to see whether any organisations you are associated with, or work for, are committed to implementing the Charter (organisations 'adopting' the Charter will be named in the leaflet). If you find your organisation has not adopted the Charter, then ask an appropriate person if they can explain that decision to you.

ACTIVITY 17

Making choices

- How does the work you do 'enable' carers to make choices? Jot down a sentence or two below.

ACTIVITY 18

Finding the right department

- Find out the full name of your local social services/social work department, including the local council that department is part of. Write down your answer below.

ACTIVITY 19

Assessment stages

- Think of any assessment that you've observed, or been part of. How many stages could you pick out in the way the assessment was put together? At what stage(s) is consultation with service users important? Use the space below to jot down your answers.

ACTIVITY 20

Finding the right kinds of help

- Could any people you are working with benefit from social services help they don't seem to be receiving? Make a note of what you think such people need, and show it to your line manager or supervisor.

ACTIVITY 21

Quality services

- You can see that the 'commissioning' of health services is getting much closer to the experience of people who actually use those services. That means there will be more people planning those services, and more variation in the services provided from area to area (depending on local needs and preferences). Can you think why 'this Government wants to see a National Health Service which offers dependable, high standards of care and treatment everywhere'? (*A First Class Service: Quality in the New NHS*, 1998). What you read about 'inequalities' in the previous section should give you a clue. Write a sentence or two below.

ACTIVITY 22

Getting well, or staying well

- Thinking about the definition above, is there a difference between helping someone get better and helping them stay well? Write a line or two below; it will help you understand a little more about some of the nursing roles outlined in the remainder of this section. Then read the quotation below ('Trust partnership gives club a real leg-up'); it's a good example of how nursing roles have come to include both getting people better and helping them stay that way.

ACTIVITY 23

Community health services

- Write a sentence or two below (or at the back of this book) picking out any services an older person in your care might benefit from but does not get at present. Show those notes to your line manager or supervisor.

ACTIVITY 24

Unclaimed benefits

- Can you think of anyone in your care who might be entitled to benefits they haven't claimed? How might you encourage them to make a claim? List some suggestions below.

ACTIVITY 25

'Whistle blowing'

- How might you feel if you had to 'blow the whistle' (ie, 'tell') on someone at work? Write a sentence or two starting 'What I would do if I found someone doing something wrong and couldn't persuade them to stop is ...'

ACTIVITY 26

Applying what you've learned

1 Write down what you knew about community care for older people and their carers before you started reading the guide.

2 Work out what you thought you would gain from reading the guide, and share this with your line manager, or someone from a carers' organisation both of you belong to.

3 In discussions with your manager, or your colleague, work out what it is you need to do differently now that you've read the guide.

4 **Wait till you've put those changes into practice, and then ask your manager, or your colleague for their honest opinion on how well you're doing.**

How well have we done?

If you remember, this book had three broad objectives (see page ix). Those objectives are:

1 To help identify all those people, 'professionals' and others, who can help you care for older people you work with.
2 To help you recognise the very important contribution you as a carer make to the caring 'team'.
3 To help you understand what services there are for older people, why they work in the way(s) they do, and what they can and cannot do.

We would like you now to make a note in your own words of how well you think this book met those objectives. Please use the box below if that helps you.

How well have we done?

- Objective 1:
- Objective 2:
- Objective 3:

References

A First Class Service: Quality in the new NHS (1998) Department of Health, London.

A Quality Strategy for Social Care (2000) Executive Summary, Department of Health, London.

About NHS Direct (2001) Department of Health, London.

Abuse Matters: A training package to meet the requirements of Unit Z1, S/NVQ in Care (1999) AEA, London.

ACAS (2000) Latest employment developments, October 2000, ACAS, London.

Age Concern Factsheet 37 (2000) *Hospital discharge arrangements and NHS continuing health care services*, Age Concern Information Line, Ashburton, Devon.

Age Concern's priorities for the next parliament (2001) Age Concern England, London.

Age discrimination in health and social care (2000) King's Fund Briefing note, London.

Alcoe J & Parker C (1987) A harsh reality, *Social Services Insight*, 16.01.87.

ANANOVA (2001) NHS 'equal treatment guarantee' for pensioners, 27.03.01. www.ananova.com

Annual Report (1998–1999) Suffolk Health Authority, Ipswich.

Annual Reports (1998/1999) Local Health Partnerships NHS Trust, Ipswich.

Banks P (1998) Carers: Making the connections, *Managing Community Care*, Vol. 6 (6): 240–245.

Barner M, Evans R, Hertzman C, and Lomas J (1982) Ageing and health care utilisation: new evidence on old fallacies, *Social Science and Medicine*, Vol. 24 (10): 851–862.

Bell L (1999) *CareFully*, 2nd Edition, Age Concern England, London.

Better Services for Vulnerable People (1998) Department of Health, EL(97)62.

Brand D (2000) User Participation in Setting and Regulating Standards for Social Care, *Managing Community Care*, Vol. 8 (4): 7–10.

Browne M (1996) Needs Assessment and Community Care, in Percy-Smith J (ed) *Needs Assessment in Public Policy*, Open University Press, Buckingham.

Carers and Disabled Children Act Summary (2001) Department of Health, London.

Carers in Employment: A report on the development of policies to support carers at work (1995) The Princess Royal Trust for Carers, London.

Caring about Carers: A National Strategy for Carers (1999) HMSO, London.

Caring for People (1989) HMSO, London.

Charging with Care: How Councils charge for home care (2000) Audit Commission, London.

Charter for Carers in Suffolk (1999) Carers Charter Group, Ipswich.

Community Care (Direct Payments) Act 1996, Draft Policy and Practice Consultation Paper (1999) Department of Health, London.

Croft P and Beresford S (1993) *Getting involved: a practical manual*, Open Services Project and Joseph Rowntree Foundation, London.

Day P and Klein R (1988) Quietly creating a revolution in community care, *The Health Service Journal*, 24.03.88.

Dow D (2000) Community Care and the Law, *Managing Community Care*, Vol. 8 (2): 9–14.

Flynn N (1990) Survival guide, *Social Services Insight*, 01.08.90.

General Household Survey (1992) *Carers in 1990*, OPCS, London.

Getting the most from your primary care team (1998) Carers National Association, London.

Grice A and Brown C (1999) Over-50's to get ensured minimum income, *The Independent*, 02.11.99, Edition No. 4069.

Guidance on the Health Act Section 31 Partnership Arrangements (2000) Department of Environment, Transport, and the Regions, Department for Education and Employment, Department of Health, London.

Guidelines for assessment and care management including NHS Continuing Care (1997) Suffolk Social Services and Suffolk Health, Ipswich.

Ham C (1991) *The New National Health Service*, Ratcliffe Medical Press, Oxford.

Henderson V (1966) *The Nature of Nursing*, Macmillan, New York.

How do I get help? A carer's guide to assessments (1999) Carers National Association, London.

Information for people with cancer and their carers (1998) East Suffolk Palliative Care Network Group, Ipswich.

Janzon K (1998) Eligibility Criteria: a Case of Muddling Through?, *Managing Community Care*, Vol. 6 (5): 209–216.

Jones N (2000) Joint Investment Plan: A Positive Move Forward, *Managing Community Care*, Vol. 8 (5): 3–5.

Kendra I (1997) National Lottery, *Community Care*, 18.12.97.

King's Fund News, London, 11 November 2000.

Laslett P (1989) *A Fresh Map of Life*, Weidenfeld and Nicolson, London.

Lewis P (2000) Blair's Blueprint For Those In Care, *Saga Magazine*, September: 143–144.

Lloyd A and Hill-Tout J (1998) NHS Trusts and Provision of Services, in Merry P (ed) 1998, *NHS Handbook*, 13th Edition, JMH Publishing, Tunbridge Wells.

Macmillan Nurses and Marie Curie Nurses, *Marie Curie News*, Winter 1998: 8–9.

Meteyard B (1994) *Community Care Keyworker Manual*, 2nd Edition, Pavilion Publishing and JICC Ltd, Brighton.

Modernising the Social Care Workforce – the first national training strategy for England (2000) Training Organisation for the Personal Social Services (TOPSS) England, Leeds.

Modernising Social Services (1998) HMSO, London, Cm. 4169.

The National Service Framework for Older People, Executive Summary (2001) Department of Health, London.

New Care Awards: Information Leaflet (1997) Local Government Management Board, London.

The New NHS Modern Dependable (1997) HMSO, London, Cm. 3807.

The New Primary Care Groups: the knowledge and skills nurses need to make them a real success (1998) Royal College of Nursing, London.

The NHS Plan (2000), The Government's response to the Royal Commission on Long Term Care, Department of Health, London.

The NHS Plan: A plan for investment; A plan for reform (2000) Department of Health, London.

Nocon A and Baldwin S (1998) *Trends in Rehabilitation Policy – A literature review*, King's Fund, London.

Nolan M and Caldock K (1996) Assessment: identifying the barriers to good practice, *Health and Social Care in the Community*, Vol. 4 (2): 77–85.

Patterson J (1999) *Disability Rights Handbook*, 24th Edition, Disability Rights Alliance, London.

Peplau H (1988) *Interpersonal Relations in Nursing*, Macmillan, Basingstoke.

Rehabilitation and intermediate care for older people (2000) King's Fund occasional briefing paper, London.

Rickford F (2000) We Will Survive, *Community Care*, 31 August–6 September: 16–18.

Robinson J (1999) Rehabilitation, *Managing Community Care*, Vol. 7 (4): 39–44.

Robinson J, Banks P, Greatley A, and Stevenson J (2000) The NHS Plan: What Does it Mean for Community Care, *Managing Community Care*, Vol. 8 (6): 5–10.

Rogers A and Elliott H (1997) *Primary Care; Understanding Health Need and Demand*, Ratcliffe Medical Press, Abingdon.

So what do social workers do? (1999) Association of Directors of Social Services, London.

Social Trends (2001) National Statistics: Social Trends, The Stationery Office, London.

Social Workers: Their Role and Tasks (1982) National Institute for Social Work, London.

Stevenson J (1999) Comprehensive Assessment of Older People, *Managing Community Care*, Vol. 7 (5): 7–14.

Suffolk Disability Information Handbook, 2nd Edition (1997) Suffolk Disability Information Group, Ipswich.

Summerskill B (2001) Fear grips old as care home closures close, *The Observer*, 25.03.01.

Thistlethwaite P (1998) Community Care at the Millennium, in *Community Care* 1999–2002, Pavilion Publishing, Brighton.

Trappes-Lomax T (1999) Messages from the Front Line: Joint Health and Social care Rehabilitation, *Managing Community Care*, Vol. 7 (4): 33–37.

Tree D (2000) Charging for Home Care Services, *Managing Community Care*, Vol. 8 (4): 3–6.

Waddington P and Filby M (1999) On Developing Primary Care Groups as Effective Organisations, *Managing Community Care*, Vol. 7 (5): 25–34.

Waugh P (1999) Homes for the old get tough new watchdog, *The Independent*, 08.09.99, Edition No. 4022.

The Way to go Home: Rehabilitation and Remedial Services for Older People (2000) Audit Commission, London.

Westland P (1988) A double-edged weapon, *Community Care*, 31.03.88.

Winkler F (1998) Primary and Community Care Services, in Merry P (ed) 1998, *NHS Handbook*, 13th Edition, JMH Publishing, Tunbridge Wells.

Wistow G et al (1994) *Social Care in a Mixed Economy*, Open University Press, Buckingham.

With Respect to Old Age: A synopsis of the Report by the Royal Commission on Long Term Care (1999) Saga Magazine, Folkestone.

Appendix 1
Useful addresses

Action on Elder Abuse
1268 London Road
London SW16 4ER
Tel: 020 8764 7648
Elder Abuse Response: 0808 808 8141 (Mon–Fri 10am–4.30pm)

Age Concern England
Astral House
1268 London Road
London SW16 4ER
Tel: 020 8765 7200
Fax: 020 8765 7211

Age Concern Cymru
4th Floor, 1 Cathedral Road
Cardiff CF1 9SD
Tel: 029 2037 1566
Fax: 029 2039 9562

Age Concern Scotland
113 Rose Street
Edinburgh EH2 3DT
Tel: 0131 220 3345
Fax: 0131 220 2779

Age Concern Northern Ireland
3 Lower Crescent
Belfast BT7 1NR
Tel: 028 9024 5729
Fax: 028 9023 5497

Alzheimer's Society
Gordon House
10 Greencoat Place
London SW1P 1PH
Tel: 020 7306 0606

Arthritis Care
18 Stephenson Way
London NW1 2HD
Tel: 020 7916 1500
Freephone: 0800 289 170 (Mon–Fri 12noon–4pm)

Benefits Agency
See your local telephone directory for the office covering your postal district; for central helplines; and for Benefit Enquiry line numbers, or visit the DSS website on http://www.dss.gov.uk

Carers National Association
20-25 Glasshouse Yard
London EC1A 4JT
Tel: 020 7490 8818
CarersLine: 0345 573 369

Carers Association Northern Ireland
113 University Street
Belfast BT7 1HP
Tel: 028 9043 9843

Carers Association Scotland
3rd Floor, 162 Buchanan Street
Glasgow G1 2LL
Tel: 0141 333 9495

Carers Association Wales
Pantglas Industrial Estate
Bedwas
Newport NP1 8DR
Tel: 029 2081 1370

Child Poverty Action Group
94 White Lion Street
London N1 9PF
Tel: 020 7837 7979

Citizens Advice Bureau
Look in local telephone directory under Citizens Advice Bureau

City and Guilds Affinity
1 Giltspur Street
London EC1A 9DD
Tel: 020 7294 2468

Community health councils/Local health councils (Scotland)
Look in local telephone directory under the name of the community health council or local health council where you live.

Contact
15 Henrietta Street
London WC2E 8HQ
Tel: 020 7240 0630

Counsel and Care
Lower Ground Floor
Twyman House
16 Bonny Street
London NW1 9PG
Tel: 020 7485 1550
Helpline: 0845 300 7585 (10.30–12.00pm and 2.00pm–4.00pm)

CRUSE – Bereavement Care
126 Sheen Road
Richmond
Surrey TW9 1UR
Tel: 020 8940 4818

Disability Alliance
Universal House
88-94 Wentworth Street
London E1 7SA
Tel: 020 7247 8765

Help the Aged
207-221 Pentonville Road
London N1 9UZ
Tel: 020 7278 1114

Jewish Women's Aid
PO Box 14270
London N12 8WG
Tel: 020 8445 8060
Freephone: 0800 591 203

National Extension College
18 Brooklands Avenue
Cambridge CB2 2HN
Tel: 01223 450300

Northern Ireland Women's Aid Federation
129 University Street
Belfast BT7 1HP
Tel: 028 9024 9041
Helpline: 028 9033 1818 (24-hour)

The Open University
Walton Hall
Milton Keynes MK7 6AA
Prospectus Request Line: 01908 858585

Parkinson's Disease Society of the UK
215 Vauxhall Bridge Road
London SW1V 1EJ
Tel: 020 7931 8080
Helpline: 020 7233 5373

Partially Sighted Society
Queen's Road
Doncaster
South Yorkshire DN1 2NX
Tel: 01302 323132

The Princess Royal Trust for Carers
142 Minories
London EC3N 1LS
Tel: 020 7480 7788

Public Concern at Work
Suite 306
16 Baldwins Gardens
London EC1N 7RT
Tel: 020 7404 6609

Relatives and Residents Association
5 Tavistock Place
London WC1H 9SN
Tel: 020 7916 6055

Royal National Institute for the Blind (RNIB)
224 Great Portland Street
London W1N 6AA
Tel: 020 7388 1266
Helpline: 0345 669999

The Royal National Institute for Deaf People (RNID)
19-23 Featherstone Street
London EC1Y 8SL
Tel: 020 7296 8000
Textphone: 020 7296 8001
Helpline: 0808 808 0123
Helpline textphone: 0808 808 9000

Scottish Women's Aid
Norton Park
57 Albion Road
Edinburgh EH7 5QY
Tel: 0131 475 2372

Social Care Association (SCA)
Thornton House
Hook Road
Surbiton
Surrey KT6 5AR
Tel: 020 8397 1411

Southall Black Sisters
52 Norwood Road
Southall UB2 4DW
Tel: 020 8571 9595

Standing Committee for Ethnic Minority Senior Citizens
5 Westminster Bridge Road
London SE1 7XW
Tel: 020 7928 0095

Unison
1 Mabledon Place
London WC1H 9AJ
Tel: 020 7388 2366

Unison Education
20 Grand Depot Road
London SE18 6SF
Tel: 020 8854 2244

Victim Support (National Office)
Cranmer House
39 Cranmer Road
London SW9 6DZ
Tel: 020 7735 9166

Victim Support Northern Ireland
Annsgate House
70-74 Ann Street
Edinburgh EH2 2HB
Tel: 0131 225 7779

Women's Aid National Office
PO Box 391
Bristol BS99 7WS
Tel: 0117 944 4411 (office)
Helpline: 0345 023 468 (24-hour)

Appendix 2
Sample letter requesting a carer's assessment

Below is a sample letter you could write to social services. The instructions in brackets refer to the information about you and the person you care for which you will need to include in your own letter. Remember that you can ask for a carer's assessment in your own right – it need not be linked to any assessment of the needs of the person you are caring for.

12 Another Road
Another Town
London SW16 4JR
Tel: 020 8865 8000

21 May 2001

Social services address

Dear Sir/Madam

I am writing on behalf of (name and address of the person you care for). S/he is my (mother, husband, friend etc). I am writing to request an assessment for community care services.

(name of person) needs help because s/he is (list here the disabilities that your friend or relative has, eg, she is 90 years old, has arthritis and is becoming frail). The main things s/he needs help with are (list here the problems your friend or relative has, eg having a bath, cleaning etc).

I am his/her carer and I would also like to request a care assessment under the Carer's Act. The main difficulties that I am having are (list here the things that you think you need, eg, I need a break from caring).

Could you please write to me at the above address or telephone me on (put your number here) to let me know when you will be able to carry out an assessment.

Yours faithfully

Jane Smith

Make a copy of your letter so that you can refer to it in future. Someone will contact you, probably a social worker. Call social services if you do not hear from them within two weeks.

If you need help urgently, you could add an extra sentence to explain the urgency. Alternatively, you might do better to telephone social services, explain the situation, and ask for their immediate help. In emergencies, social services can provide services before carrying out a full assessment. Don't forget that under the Carers and Disabled Children Act 2000 you can request an assessment independently of the person you are caring for. You can even ask for an assessment if that person has refused an assessment themselves.

(Source: *How do I get help?*, Carers National Association)

About Age Concern

An Introductory Guide to Community Care is one of a wide range of publications produced by Age Concern England, the National Council on Ageing. Age Concern works on behalf of all older people and believes later life should be fulfilling and enjoyable. For too many this is impossible. As the leading charitable movement in the UK concerned with ageing and older people, Age Concern finds effective ways to change that situation.

Where possible, we enable older people to solve problems themselves, providing as much or as little support as they need. A network of local Age Concerns, supported by 250,000 volunteers, provides community-based services such as lunch clubs, day centres and home visiting.

Nationally, we take a lead role in campaigning, parliamentary work, policy analysis, research, specialist information and advice provision, and publishing. Innovative programmes promote healthier lifestyles and provide older people with opportunities to give the experience of a lifetime back to their communities.

Age Concern is dependent on donations, covenants and legacies.

Age Concern England
1268 London Road
London SW16 4ER
Tel: 020 8765 7200
Fax: 020 8765 7211

Age Concern Cymru
4th Floor
1 Cathedral Road
Cardiff CF1 9SD
Tel: 029 2037 1566
Fax: 029 2039 9562

Age Concern Scotland
113 Rose Street
Edinburgh EH2 3DT
Tel: 0131 220 3345
Fax: 0131 220 2779

Age Concern Northern Ireland
3 Lower Crescent
Belfast BT7 1NR
Tel: 028 9024 5729
Fax: 028 9023 5497

Publications from Age Concern Books

Promoting Mobility for People with Dementia: A problem-solving approach
Rosemary Oddy

People with dementia must be encouraged and enabled to move and given the opportunity to do so frequently, with or without help, if they are to remain mobile. This new book outlines commonsense approaches to ease this task and help to maintain optimum levels of mobility for people with dementia for as long as possible, without jeopardising the health and safety of those who care for them.

Throughout this book many of the problems associated with mobility are identified and suggestions made on how to ease or overcome them. Finding ways of communicating effectively in order to promote movement is central to the approach, as is the importance of planning ahead. Based on years of experience, this book contains a wealth of fresh and practical suggestions for physiotherapists, occupational therapists, nurses and carers.

£14.99 0-86242-242-6

CareFully: A handbook for home care assistants, 2nd Edition
Lesley Bell

Comprehensive and informative, this new edition of a highly acclaimed guide provides key advice for home care workers in promoting independence. Packed with practical guidance, detailed information on good practice and recent developments in home care provision, all chapters are related to S/NVQ Level 2 revised units in care. Topics covered in full include:

- basic skills of home care assistants
- the health of older people
- receiving home care – the user perspective

- the importance of core values
- providing a service for the new millennium
- taking care of yourself

£12.99 0-86242-285-X

Age Concern Training Packs

Age Concern Training Packs are ideal teaching tools for all care staff involved in the training and support of other staff. They enable trainers to effectively guide and reinforce skills and development by providing all the material necessary to run successful group training sessions.

The Training Packs:

- can be used either as an integrated or topic-led course
- can be used again and again
- can be used by inexperienced trainers
- save time and money

All contain key point overhead transparencies, aims and objectives, teaching plans, group activities and support material and handouts.

Accident Prevention in Residential and Nursing Homes: A training pack
Royal Society for the Prevention of Accidents (RoSPA)

For older people living in residential and nursing homes, the move into unfamiliar territory is often associated with accidents involving injuries. With people living longer and becoming more frail, the burden of responsibility of care staff is steadily increasing. This pack supports managers, supervisors and carers in achieving the highest standards of safety by providing training material on:

- the effects of ageing
- the responsibility for home safety
- the types of accidents experienced by older people
- falls and older people
- risk assessment
- maintaining a safe environment

Based on RoSPA safety training seminars, this training material provides key point overhead transparencies, summaries, aims and objectives and recommended time-scales in order to support all care home staff towards the development of good practice in accident prevention.

£45.00 0-86242-290-6

The Reminiscence Trainer's Pack
For use in health, housing, social care and arts organisations; colleges, libraries and museums; volunteers' and carers' agencies
Faith Gibson

This teaching pack is designed as a straightforward teaching tool to assist trainers present the basic ideas underlying planned reminiscence work which may be undertaken by a wide variety of health and social care staff, housing, library and museum staff, teachers, artists, volunteers, students and family carers.

The pack aims to equip trainers in a variety of settings, sectors and service agencies primarily concerned with older people. The training is designed to introduce reminiscence workers to the theory and practice and topics include:

- what is reminiscence?
- working with people from different cultures
- working with people with hearing, sight and speech difficulties
- working with people with dementia

Whether you are a professional carer or a family carer, reminiscence can enrich relationships and enhance caring. Containing 26 key point overhead transparencies, together with summaries, clear aims and objectives and handouts, this pack will enable the trainer to effectively guide and reinforce staff skills and development.

£35.00 0-86242-305-8

If you would like to order any of these titles, please write to the address below, enclosing a cheque or money order for the appropriate amount (plus £1.95 p&p) made payable to Age Concern England. Credit card orders may be made on 0870 44 22 044 (for individuals); or 0870 44 22 120 (AC federation, other organisations and institutions). Fax: 01626 323318

Age Concern Books
PO Box 232
Newton Abbot
Devon TQ12 4XQ

Age Concern Information Line/Factsheets subscription

Age Concern produces 44 comprehensive factsheets designed to answer many of the questions older people (or those advising them) may have. These include money and benefits, health, community care, leisure and education, and housing. For up to five free factsheets, telephone: 0800 00 99 66 (7am-7pm, seven days a week, every day of the year). Alternatively you may prefer to write to Age Concern, FREEPOST (SWB 30375), ASHBURTON, Devon TQ13 7ZZ.

For professionals working with older people, the factsheets are available on an annual subscription service, which includes updates throughout the year. For further details and costs of the subscription, please write to Age Concern at the above Freepost address.

Index